The Communication Soul-ution, Empowered Interactions

Tamara Dorris

Dedicated to the memory of my dear friend Cheryl ("Missy") who I am sure is busy flying with angels this very moment

Foreword

When I was a middle school teacher, meaningful quotes adorned my classroom walls. A favorite of mine was, "In the classroom, it's all about relationships." As my career steered me toward higher education as a professor and into business as an owner and investor, I quickly realized that *life* if about relationships. At the heart of those relationships is effective communication.

My communication skills can definitely be improved, which led me to Tamara Dorris' most recent book, *The Communication Soul-ution Empowered Interactions.* As a woman, I possess the intuition and care that Tamara discusses. However, having a father who took me under his wing as the boy he never had, I also have an aggressive, short-tempered urge to often tell it like it is. Don't ask me if you look fat in those jeans; I'll tell you the truth. My husband jokes with me that I need a filter between my brain and my mouth. Thanks to time and valuable lessons like those I've learned in *The Communication Soul-ution,*, that filter is growing daily.

Tamara begins with insight into why people communicate as they do, then provides a means of balancing our need to be right with the ultimate goal – to reach an outcome with which everyone feels comfortable. Her strategies are applicable in just about every situation imaginable. "It's Time to Talk," reinforces ways I can better communicate with and listen to my husband. "Did You Hear That?" reminds me of the elements of communication that will most effectively help me grow my business and keep my current clients coming back for more. I know that after reading *The Communication Soul-ution*, not only will my husband and clients see a new side of me, but so will my university students, children, and friends. Maybe even my mother-in-law.

As Tamara explains, real communication skills are not taught in schools. They are developed through trial and error, making some huge mistakes, and seeking forgiveness afterwards. How to effectively communicate for win-win outcomes does not have to be a mystery nor a struggle. With books such as *The Communication Soul-ution*, written in a lively, easy-to-read style, we can cut down on our mistakes and find resolutions with less mess in between. Tamara's bigger picture of communication goes beyond the spoken word and beyond the obvious. It is a much needed life tool, and now a prized addition to my library.

Dr. Shannon Maveety
T.E.A.M. Ed. Services

Table of Contents

Preface

You're holding in your hands a small book that can change your life for the better. In a nutshell, I am convinced (and I don't think anyone could debate the idea) that the majority of our happiness and success is directly and intimately related to our relationships. The way we communicate with others either delivers us right to our goals or drives us farther from them.

And this idea is not only applicable to close relationships, but to those often brief, albeit sometimes meaningful, encounters we have with complete strangers. From the guy who cuts you off at the freeway onramp, to the one who flips your burgers at the drive thru or cleans your house or sets up meetings or even changes the oil in your car. Interactions are everywhere.

When I first had friends and endorsers review this book, I got a lot of feed back that informed me, ever so graciously, that I had misspelled "Solutions." It was no accident. *"Communication Soul-utions"* is quite intentional.

This is a small book on purpose. There aren't zillions of pages to pretend to read. Everything is simplified and pared down to the bare essentials so that everyone, even those beloved communication students of mine who would rather eat tree bark than read another communications book, can wade through it with ease. Also, please note that there are numerous exercises within these pages. These exercises and questions are all about you. They are opportunities for you to honestly and constructively assess where you are and how you might improve. Do these exercises. Whether you write directly in the book or you jot your responses in a journal; it's quite critical to your ultimate success that you understand all you can about yourself.

With that, I wish you well, and hope all your interactions are soulful and empowered.

Tamara Dorris

The Communication Soul-ution, Empowered Interactions

Phoenix, Lady
for a special lady
& Spiritual Sister —
Bless you now
& always —

Empowered Press Publishing, www.empoweredpress.org
2005

Chapter One
THE WAY WE ARE

WOMEN and men communicate differently. This doesn't mean that one is better than the other. What it does mean is that we are in a state of grace, in a time when balance from both sides is required for personal growth and global recovery. The majority of communication books on the market today focus primarily on a male audience, with a business focus. Or, those publications that do target women tend to try and teach us how to get along in a big boy's world rather than accepting and improving our own natural attributes. The true secret to effective communications is combining corporate speak with intuitive introspect, candor with common sense, softness with sincerity, and honesty with integrity. This is a book about getting along better with others so that we can elevate ourselves and bring more balance into the world.

Striking balance takes energy and effort. However, it is an investment we can't afford not to make. Generally speaking, it is easier for females to hone their communication skills more masterfully than men because we inherently possess the most crucial quality: compassion. Even more important, it has come time that as a civilization we must, regardless of gender, religion or ethnicity, learn to communicate in a language that is universal. That said-- this is not a book about how women bare their souls and men grunt in response. Instead, it is a proactive interaction guide that works toward understanding self and the people in our lives more effectively, intuitively, and lovingly. These are real life rules that are simple and profound and can make your interactions effortless, stress-less and productive to your ultimate goals in life. In order to evolve on a global level we need to start within our own skin. Starting from within means that we strive to know our self and others beyond the simple surface. People need other people just to get along in the business of life.

Miscommunication is a malady that often hits us hard. Due to our generally congenial nature, women don't traditionally do very well with confrontational or conflicting communications. And that's okay. The truth is that confrontational and conflicting communications shouldn't be something any of us need to tend to very often, or at the very least, they should be something we can elegantly and assertively work around. Unfortunately, there are some individuals who might try and undermine our efforts because we are female. There are ways to work around all communication complications, even if it means leaving the room or hanging up the phone. Hopefully, it rarely needs to come to that.

Problems in our interactions generally arise from miscommunications. By definition, miscommunication is simply information that somehow becomes skewed between the speaker's mouth and the listener's ear—but a troubling outcome hits us where we live, both personally and professionally. Becoming effective in spite of the roadblocks that stand in the way is only one of the benefits you are about to receive.

In addition to overcoming conflicted communications at home and at work, our interactions can help us to attain our goals. When you understand human nature and how it operates in the overall scheme of things, you will find yourself well armed with the ammunition needed for gaining the support and assistance of others. Securing your place and standing your ground become much easier when you learn to put other people on your side. Nearly everything you do in your life, or aspire to do, from work; to love; to family; to hobbies; to dreams, will require the assistance or compliance of someone else, usually lots of someone elses.

Unless you are a hermit, living in the hills somewhere (at which point one would wonder why you're reading a book about communications), you will benefit by learning the important interaction skills that no one ever taught you in school. But they should have.

With the final destination well in mind (getting along better with anyone, living your life on purpose, and brining better energy into the world), let's take a look at the journey ahead.

GENDER DIFFERENCES is a logical place to start. This smallish chapter is dedicated to revealing the differences between the sexes, and then we move to higher ground. The reason men and women interact differently can be largely attributed to the sex-roles we encountered when we were young. Most common factors involved child rearing, education, and assertiveness. On a more positive note, women possess much stronger intuition skills then our male counterparts, which can cause us the wisdom to run companies, households, and nations. Once we've gotten the difference between genders out of the way, we'll jump right into the heart of the matter: why we say what we do and how to say it better.

In WHY OUR WORDS MATTER, we look at the ways in which nearly everything we say or do in this world has some kind of cosmic impact, even if we can't instantly spot it. The words we utter to others truly matter and when we use words that don't work *for* us, they work *against* us. Combative communications, any way you cut it, are not productive; they feel lousy, and cause stress. Stress can kill you. Simply put, there are two possible outcomes to most interactions: productive and non-productive. These outcomes are usually a result of the way in which we communicate: reactive or responsive. One is negative and the other is correct.

NEGATIVE REACTION covers the cause of non-productive communications. There are three primary topics that fall under the heading of negative reaction: THE NEED TO BE RIGHT, DEFENSIVENESS, and JUDGING. Each one of these is nothing more or nothing less than our egos and insecurities standing up and shouting loudly for the rest of the world to hear. You'll recognize the damage that an overactive ego can cause and the destruction uncalled for defensiveness wreaks. Most importantly, you'll participate in exercises that will help you identify the areas in your own life that might require attention. We'll look at eliminating negative elements in your individual interactions, as well as overcoming them when they crop up in others.

WHEN YOUR WORDS FAIL YOU unlocks the remaining components of what not to say and do in order to be your most effective. Before we can unleash our authentic power, we must first get clear on what kinds of things deplete us and why. Interrupting, yelling, and losing your cool are redefined in ways you might not usually think of, harness these and you are ready to evolve.

EFFECTIVELY YOURS, introduces you to the premise of the new theory that will teach you to respond instead of react, productively instead of not. The groundwork will be laid by touching on the important points of understanding your audience, minding your attitude, and honoring ethics and honesty in your communications with others. Minding your attitude involves a heartfelt look at depression and optimism and how each can and *do* affect every interaction you're involved in.

GOALS ARE GOLD is the first step to putting your plan into action. Here we learn why identifying our goals is paramount to improved interactions. It may sound crazy, but nothing could be closer to the truth...our goals command our communications. Every interaction has one to three goals attached to it. Once we understand that goal attainment intertwines with and around the relationships we have with other people, it becomes easier to implement change. We will look at the different levels of our interaction goals and how to instantly apply them.

STEPPING OUT on the town with your tongue in check. This is the second step in the Effective Response Theory. "Stepping Out" refers to the act of literally removing your feelings and eliminating your emotions from the interaction at hand and simply regarding the facts. When we look at the facts, less the baggage that usually attaches itself to the facts, it's amazing how different things appear. Once we see through the barrage of emotions that often cloud our communications, it's amazing how simple things can be. Perhaps it is our innate nature to reason and wonder and worry about things we should simply let go of.

Think about being in high school and spending an hour on the telephone with your girlfriend trying to analyze what someone said, even if it was only a sentence or two. Women from quilting circles to Tupperware parties have traditionally tended to gossip and gab and overanalyze anything and anyone that comes to mind.

When we get to the meat of the matter, reciting only the facts, sometimes a foggy day becomes suddenly clear.

PUT ON YOUR WALKIN' SHOES and dance. This step is about empathy. Your grandmother might have been the one to tell you not to judge someone until you've walked a mile in her shoes, and that's what we'll do here. Sometimes the other person's shoes might fit so tight we get blisters, and other times, there's enough room to wiggle our toes. The point is that empathy is an asset, and gratefully, one that comes easy for most of us.

When we make an effort to understand the space or place someone else is working from, we become empowered to make a monumental difference in what we say next. Empathy allows us to heal hearts, feed hungry children, mend broken nations and talk to one another more openly and caring.

ASK FOR AN ANSWER, but make the question good. How can we learn what other people want if we don't ask them? Learn to ask questions that work and construct your communications in a way that tells you what you need to know. There are different kinds of questions that provide you with different kinds of answers, and knowing what they are will help you become better at interacting with others.

Besides asking questions of others, perhaps the most important kinds of questions we can ask are those we ask of ourselves. When we question our self, our motives, and our reasons for doing or saying the things we do, we open up our hearts to hear the truth. If we answer honestly, we find out things about us that we never knew before.

DID YOU HEAR THAT? After you ask questions, you've got to listen. Listening is by far one of the toughest communication skills to adopt. We work so hard on perfecting our speaking and presentation skills that we often overlook this critical component. What an enormous mistake. People need to be heard so they can be validated. When we listen to what someone says, we validate that person. Nothing all that difficult, yet many of us fail terribly both at work and home.

Listening doesn't only meaning hearing with your ears. It means absorbing with your body the things that someone is telling you, the points they are making and the thoughts they are sharing. Moreover, you have to learn to hear what's *not* being said. Sometimes, people don't say what they mean, or they might not even know what they mean. When this happens, it's important to pay attention to clues and cues that will help you to respond. Reading body language, using the feedback tool, and understanding the art of silence will be of great benefit.

IT'S TIME TO TALK, so pull up a chair and let's have a chat. Now we take the steps of the Effective Response Theory and try them on for size. When it's time to respond (instead of react), we remain calm, maintain good eye contact, use productive words and gestures, and speak with genuine confidence, secure in ourselves and in our efforts.

When we fail to keep calm, bad things can happen. Our stress level might sky-rocket to the moon, we feel bad, and we probably cause those around us to feel even worse. Shame on us. Don't lose your cool and don't allow others to lose their cool with you. Walk away, breathe, and take a minute to think things over.

There are ways we use our words that are good and ways we use them that are not. For instance, the word "you" can be used beautifully when you're giving credit or credence to the other person. However, that same word can wound when you use it at the beginning of a confrontational communication. Be careful with your words; they mend fences or burn bridges.

The way you move your body says a lot about who you are. Sometimes, it means even more than the words you say, so pay attention to the lingo. Learn what certain gestures mean and make sure they're the messages you want to send. Use your body in a way that makes you more effective. Don't use it as a weapon; it's a gift.

Learn how to build instant rapport, deliver bad news in the best possible way, and overlook insecurity in others when you speak. This is not only effective communications, it is effective living. We will examine these techniques applied in real time by applying them to a "Before and After" interaction scenario. Here you will again be asked to participate in a series of exercises that will test your knowledge and explore your own mystique more deeply. By now you will have undoubtedly picked up some interaction savvy, and the exercises here will give you a chance to show it off.

IT'S ABOUT BEING NICE and we all should know it by now, but sadly, we do not. In a world often wrought with hysteria, fear and hate, it's not always easy to be nice. But it's important. With high pressure, late bills, and cars that break down in the rain, it's often easy to forget who we are because we're so busy being the part of us we're trying hard to change. Being nice involves some very special traits that will help you evolve as a woman and kindred spirit who is trying to do her part to heal the world. Getting along with others is the best place to start.

Chapter Two
GENDER DIFFERENCES

IT IS IMPORTANT to understand from the beginning that the main premise of this book is universal in gender. Anyone can improve his or her communication skills by following these techniques, and everyone will need to for genuine harmony and global healing to take place. There are universal truths that can and should be applied by everyone. However, because this book is geared toward a female audience, you will find parts that are very gender specific. That said the hope is that we teach, by example, our sons, husbands, brothers and fathers the truly "new" and necessary means of human interaction. It can still mean big business deals, climbing corporate ladders, running businesses and running for office, if that's what you want it to mean. It doesn't matter who you are, what your sexual preference is, or what you had for dinner last night; all we care about here is learning to get along better with others and living life on purpose.

Now that we understand these techniques are timeless and universal, let's get the prevalent gender differences out of the way. We are all beings comprised of energy and ego, love and light. We all need and want love and acceptance. There are, however, some primary differences between the genders that directly impact our communication efforts. The sooner we bring those to light the quicker we can get to the business at hand. Women and men have always been treated differently; this is no national secret. Let's touch on a few of the areas that are most obvious in an effort to level the playing field and get off to an even start. Childrearing, education, assertiveness and intuition tend to be the components that contribute most greatly to our gender difference identity, hence, play a role in the role we play in the world as women.

Let's face it: boys and girls are raised differently. Regardless of how much we try to bring about a sense of equality, nary a father fails to get his tail feathers tangled if his son receives an Easy-Bake oven or Barbie Doll for his birthday. While it's okay for girls to get trucks and play basketball (even this took eons), there is still a social stigma to the feminine side of the masculine male, and that's how it's always been. But shouldn't be.

When we were little girls, pretty and pink and stomping our feet when we wanted our way, we were developing manipulative communication skills. Meanwhile, our brothers were learning how to blow up bullfrogs with firecrackers, and to bow their head in fake remorse when captured by a grown-up. We learned to say we were sorry if we so much as spilled a drop of milk on our dry clean only dress, while our brother could wear his lunch on his shirt and no one thought a thing about it. In essence, we were raised like different species.

If you consider the vast chasm that existed in raising boys vs. girls, it doesn't take a rocket scientist to figure out that the way we would eventually grow up, think about our self, make our way in the world, and talk to other people, would vary just as dramatically. All of these differences resulted in a host of communication faux pas for both parties: boys didn't say it softly, or didn't say it at all, while women said too much, and tried to fill the role of "pretty little people pleaser."

In their book <u>More Power To You,</u> Connie Brown Glaser and Barbara Steinberg Smalley talk about women in corporate communications. They note the childhood gender differences, which are easy to identify in adulthood:

"Little girls are reluctant to complain; avoid confrontation," while boys, "state grievances directly." They go on to say that females have thin skin, and males, thick skin; girls are emotional under pressure, men cool; females hold more grudges, men hold less.
Consider the messages we are sent when we are young and it becomes easy to understand how both genders have difficulty interacting with those of the opposite and of the same sex.

We can't change the way we grew up. What we can change is the way we raise our own children, and in doing so, at least have an impact on the way they raise theirs. What we can do is identify and acknowledge that the way we were raised played a key role in the way we communicate as grown ups, which sometimes probably doesn't feel very grown up at all.

Even if we were blessed with caretakers who celebrated universal thinking and prompted the feminine and masculine qualities in children of both sexes, society at large would soon enough erase the good and reverse the effort.

As if the home front wasn't contrary enough training, we have the educational system to thank. Historically, boys have had the brains and girls could learn English and how to type. While efforts continue to evolve, our learning system still contributes greatly to the inequities of children, hence, the way they ultimately learn to communicate with the world at large.

In *Education Gender Gaps,* written by the American Association of University Women's Education Foundation and researched by the America Institution for Research,
"In 1992 *How Schools Short Change Girls,* reported serious inequities in our nations classrooms. The authors found that 1) girls received less teacher attention than boys; 2) girls received less complex and challenging interaction with their teachers than boys; 3) girls received less constructive feedback from their teachers than boys; and, 4) gender bias in teacher-student interaction in math and science showed the largest inequities.

The combination of home and school inequitable treatment contributed greatly to the third notable difference between men and women and the way they communicate. Men are simply more assertive than women. Understand that assertiveness in this context is born of self-esteem. And why wouldn't they be more assertive? If they were favored at home, in school, and in society at large, would it be any wonder that they might pack a little more power when it comes to confidence? Of course not.

In, *How to be an Assertive Woman,* Jean Baer says, "Since childhood women have been trained to hold back and control their negative feelings. The admonitions come early on: "Forgive and forget:..."Not to Care"..."Someone has to keep peace in the family"...Talk about it when you've cooled off" ..."Nice girls don't get into fights." Unfortunately, the price we've paid for swallowing our assertive tendencies has been terribly high. When we learn to trust ourselves and speak with honor and learn to respect everyone around us, assertiveness comes easy.

Please keep in mind that it is not our purpose here to point fingers or demand recourse. That is another issue, a different book. Instead, we are going to learn how to reach our goals by learning how to play nice with everyone: both genders, at home, at work, in church and at the grocery store. First though, we've got to look at why we are the way we are so we can understand that it has taken centuries of conditioning to get here; it might take a few more minutes to turn things around.

Finally, and to our favor, the last gender communication difference we will discuss is intuition. Intuition is that small voice inside your head and heart that tells you things you otherwise wouldn't know. Many successful executives (both male and female) have learned to harness and use this power effectively. Intuition, however, is inherent and apparent more strongly in the female gender, hence the term "female intuition." This is supported in *In Games Mother Never Taught You,* by Betty Lahh Harrigan, "The universal male reliance is in the power of logical thinking." Although general in statement, men tend to be left-brained, which is primarily analytical thinking (math and science), whereas females tend to be right-brained, more creative and spatial in thought.

The right-brained thinker, by default, is generally more sensitive, passionate, creative, and intuitive. This is why even men usually find more comfort and support in their female friends versus their male ones. A women's intuition is a great power, yet make no mistake, again it is critical for both genders to strike balance. So while our male counter parts must learn to adopt a more compassionate and creative way to communicate, we too should continually strive to sharpen our skills and continue to grow.

Let's assume, or at least imagine with positive intent, that the cards are stacked evenly, that the men and women and children of this world are equally and mutually respectful of one another, and that we may get on with the business of getting along.

Chapter Three
WHY OUR WORDS MATTER

ARE you ready to change your life? If you are, you've picked a fine place to start. There is no greater effort or contribution you could make toward your life and the lives of others than to learn (and teach) improved interactions. Getting along better with others does not require a magic potion; however, once you understand and apply the power of your words, nothing short of magic will occur. The techniques you are about to read are fail-proof. If you apply these strategies, you will be that much closer to achieving your goals, both personally and professionally, and ultimately globally. The words you utter make a difference in this world.

Whether it is an opportunity to assert yourself in a positive manner, comfort a child, inspire a partner or friend, ask for a raise or negotiate a contract, your words count, and learning to use them more productively will change your life forever (and other lives untold).

Abraham Maslow talked about self-realization. In his Pyramid of Human Needs, the Master himself noted that the need to be liked and accepted by others was a pretty big priority for most people.

We need other people and they need us. We need to feel loved and wanted, accepted and validated. We need to relate to other human beings for our very survival. It's not possible to progress on this planet without the assistance and compliance of others. Whether we want someone to hire us, marry us, check our bags at the airport, sell us a house, bring us food, or sign on the dotted line; other people are vital to our success. The realization that we need other people is perhaps the first step toward improved interactions. Moreover, our human evolution depends on our increased ability to work better with one another.

As women, one of our biggest downfalls tends to be the fact that we let things bother us when they shouldn't. If a cab driver is rude, even after you've applied the techniques you're about to learn to the best of your ability, then write the cabbie off as a jerk and don't ride with him again. Learning to let go of these smaller and more rare instances will become easier once you recognize how much power and control you *do* have over the majority of your interactions and the positive affect you bring to the world.

Accepting how important others are to our personal and professional happiness helps us understand why it is so important to make special efforts to improve those relationships. All of our relationships are maintained or improved or worsened by the things we say and the way we say them. This book is about keeping those relationships positive and productive.

When we fail to maintain positive relationships, it affects our personal universe.

For example, if you have a heated argument with your partner before you leave for work, chances are that you will start your workday in a negative state of mind. You might flash on the argument throughout the day, causing your blood pressure to soar or your mood to be irritable. Or, you might sink into a sullen depression, not feeling quite up to anything that requires your energy or attention. Likewise, if you've had a bad day at work, say an argument with a co-worker, you might find that you take it home with you, snapping at someone you love over dinner. These are two common examples that we all can relate to, but shouldn't have to.

If you follow these techniques with honest earnest effort you will notice empathy enters your interactions more than before. You will begin to feel aware when challenging conversations surface, and then a light inside yourself when you successfully elude them. A new vitality consumes you. It is easy to see, as in the examples above, why our interactions are an important part of our daily life. When we learn to effectively interact with others, we avoid some of the communication conflicts and pitfalls that cause us pain, problems, and prolonged frustration. We cannot go far when we feel bad. When we have heated arguments and negative confrontations, we feel bad. But this is just the beginning.

If you are trying to close a sale, motivate an employee, inspire a young person or confront your mother, what you say and how you say it are the keys to your success. Here then, we are not talking about communicating as only a way to avoid conflict, but as a way to accomplish a goal. Almost everything we do in life involves interaction with others. Logically then, our communications impact everything from the goals we set for ourselves to our physical well-being. Yes, our physical well-being.

In his book, *Learned Optimism,* Dr. Seligman tells us, "There is convincing evidence that psychological states do affect your health." In numerous studies, negativity and depression have been proven to cause disease and depression. They might even make us die younger. It's easy enough to differentiate depression or stress from communications, but have you considered the relationship?

Think about the last time you became upset or angry. Chances are at least one other person had something to do with it, yes? These are only a few things that come to mind: betrayal, screaming children, overdue reports, late bills, mean bosses, a fender bender at a stop sign, or maybe a fight with your significant other. These examples are far ranging enough that anyone should be able to find one that sticks. Notice though, that each one involves *another person* that you need to contend with in order to resolve the issue. Whether it is a partner, a prankster, or a bill collector, someone will stand before you. And it's someone you'll need to interact with—how will things unfold?

When we are already in a state of anxiety our interactions are automatically heated. Our blood pressure rages, our heart pounds, and we may even get shaky in the knees. How can we communicate effectively when our body feels like it's falling apart? When we feel that we have no control over the situation, we tend to become even more agitated. Regardless of how the interaction might end, one thing is certain: if we allowed ourselves to get angry, upset, or out of control, we have lost, regardless of the outcome.

It is important to note that men traditionally and generally handle stress and arguments differently than women. It's not a bad thing that the female gender is often more sensitive than her male counterpart. It is, however, a bad thing when we don't recognize and learn to work with these sensitivities in a way that best behoove us. When we try to overlook an upsetting confrontation, we tend to "stuff" it down our throats with ice cream or burritos, shopping trips we can't afford to take, or some other equally unproductive activity that helps us forget we're female. It would be better to remember. And then to realign.

Yes, the differences between the genders should be recognized . and reckoned with in a manner that benefits both, but the best place you can start is with yourself. Don't let a negative interactions cause you stress, worry, or depression.

Some of the female diseases that can be directly related to stress are: eating disorders/obesity, irritable bowel syndrome, heart disease and heart attack, high cholesterol, and diabetes. Not a menu any of us would like to eat from.

The point to glean is that the way we communicate, or sometimes fail to communicate, has a very definite impact on our attitudes, emotions, mood, and health. And, as Dr. Seligman has aptly pointed out, a little bad goes a long way. Since our interactions with others consume such a large part of our daily lives, it is vital that we recognize the affect that our communications have on our minds, bodies, and attitudes. We are what we speak—listen closely.

Our competitive nature being what it is, we often overlook the original intent behind our communications. When this happens, it is not unusual for us to get caught up in the battle of wits and reason and fail to accomplish our mission. Consider the following example:

If you are at a restaurant, waiting to be seated and you notice another couple is seated before you, what do you do? Many of us assume an indignant air and ever so politely "correct" the hostess who did the seating. More than ever though, it is those times when we feel that we have been wronged, that we stand up on our self righteous soap boxes, ranting and raving so that all the world can see what fools we are.

Considering the example above, understand that there are two ways to communicate. That's it. No long-winded matrix filled with many varying options and "what-if's," but rather, two ways: *productive* and *non-productive*. Productive is positive and non-productive is negative. Every time you open your mouth to say something to someone else, ask yourself first, *is this going to be productive?*

If you find that you haven't been seated in the restaurant, you have to ask yourself what it is you want from the hostess. She can't undo the fact that she already seated a couple before you, so what do you want? To be seated next? Do you want something else? Do you expect an even better seat for your inconvenience? Have you *really* been inconvenienced? What if the people before you called in for reservations and you didn't? Have you considered all the angles, or did your anger and emotions take over?

Productive communications are **positive**
Non-productive communications are **negative.**

Let's look at another example of how productive communications work to help us improve an outcome. Say you need to book a flight to Chicago for an important business meeting. You call the airlines and are informed that all flights are booked. To be unproductive, all you need to do is shout at the attendant on the telephone, tell her how important your meeting is and insist on the next available flight. Chances are good that the only thing you will get is an ulcer.

When you communicate productively, you might be surprised to hear the very helpful attendant inform you which flights have the shortest standby lists, or perhaps, even explore a re-routing possibility that will get you to your meeting on time.

Understanding the two models of communications, productive and non-productive, will be paramount to your success and eventual enlightenment. You can learn to be productive all the time, with everyone you talk to. When you're interactions are productive, you stop wasting energy on useless endeavors, and dedicate your effort to more meaningful pursuits.

The purpose here is to demonstrate how important daily interactions are to your overall success, and then lead you through the steps to get there quickly. The instructions that await you will help to ensure that you reach your goals and learn to positively affect the outcomes you share with others. Simply put, we can be the women we are and still get ahead and get along well with others. We can reach our goals by improved interactions. When we reach our goals, we feel good about our self and our life, and then we can teach others the same.

On the opposite side, however, when our interactions are not productive, we get stressed, angry, and impatient. All of these emotions equal negative attitudes and increased likelihood of stress-induced poor health. It doesn't take much to imagine the overall impact all of that negativity has on our planet (or our person); just turn on the evening news.

We are what we speak so say it softly

Let's break this journey down into parts that are easy to digest. We'll swallow one section at a time, giving ourselves things to work on and think about each day. Ultimately, we will learn how to apply these practices instantly and intelligently. When every interaction leaves us feeling warm and wonderful because we know we did our best, we will truly understand the art of effective communications.

Even though life can deliver unpleasant and even painful situations, such as divorce, termination, or confrontations of any sort, you will still be one step ahead of the game if you learn the right way to work with others in your communications. The important thing to remember, regardless of how negative the situation may be, is that losing your head, screaming, calling attention to your lack of control, rarely, if ever, improves the situation. Self-control becomes much more manageable when we learn to *respond* rather than *react*. Often this is easier for women then it is for men.

This relates back to the female-sensitivity issue. Women are more inclined to sob or shop when they face an uncomfortable or disheartening confrontation. Men, on the other hand, will generally learn to maintain their composure, however, only long enough to go home and kick the dog or yell so loud it scares the neighbors. The goal here is not to sob, shout, or kick dogs; it is instead, learning to say what you need to say in a way that is conducive to the most effective outcome. You will find that once you learn the power behind these techniques, you are one hundred times more in control of yourself and the outcome than you ever thought possible

When we all learn to operate from a higher place of peace, harmony, and respect, the results will be staggering. Once we realize the power of our words, we can stop using them to hurt and start using them to heal.

Chapter Four
NEGATIVE REACTION

A SPOONFUL of medicine makes the sugar seem much sweeter. Put another way, in order to improve our interactions from a positive perspective, we must first explore what ruins them in the first place. Negative reaction is the mode many of us use to communicate in. Unless you are a monk, living in the outer regions of India, chanting mantras and sipping herbal tea each day, you probably run across people and situations that irritate you. When you get irritated or upset it isn't always easy to act like a monk, is it? Here we will examine the beasts that drive negative communications, cause wars, and ruin relationships.

One our biggest faux pas as female communicators has to do with the "cold shoulder routine." This routine is outdated, overused, and keeps us in the days of yore.

If something or someone upsets you, betrays you or embarrasses you, there are ways to deal with it effectively that we will discuss throughout this book. However, simply turning to an Ice Princess in hopes of gaining attention or pity does not take the female gender to the next level, but instead keeps it aligned with the "cave-man mentality," which does no one any good. Understand that giving someone the cold shoulder seldom, if ever, accomplishes anything genuine, beyond amusing or annoying those we are freezing out. Ignoring a person because you are hurt or angry is not effective communications; it is reacting to emotion. And it is useless.

It is our human nature to *react* rather than *respond* when we don't like what's said or done. Before we can begin to identify the beauty of the Effective Response Theory, we must first take a walk on the dark side, and it may not be so easy. When we start to understand what we do wrong (from centuries of incorrect programming and conditioning), we can learn to stop doing it. We can begin to grow and nurture our interactions through genuinely effective efforts.

To negatively react is to say the first thing that pops into your mind, often overlooking the impact your words or actions might have on the outcome of the situation or the person on the other end. For example, how many of us have shouted at a child in *reaction*, only to feel guilty later on? We feel guilty after the fact because we realize that shouting was not productive nor warranted, no matter how clumsy, thoughtless, or wild the child might have been. Thinking of everyone you come into contact with as a child is actually a good idea and has provided many people the extra patience they needed when angry emotions approach. But to delve further, let's look at what happens to us that makes us want to blow up in the first place.

There are three parts of negative reactions that we will explore, each concerning the ego. The first is known as "The Need to Be Right," and the second is "Judging," and the third, "Defensive Behavior." The lines between them are often thin, particularly because they all pertain to our ego minds, otherwise known as "me-me-me." The differences, however, are distinct enough to qualify for separate discussions. Understanding these facets of human nature will take us infinitely farther in our quest for improved interactions for two reasons.

The first and foremost benefit we can gain from self-exploration is self-discovery. If we can begin to understand how our own ego fuels our negative attitudes we can begin to control the way we interact with others. When we understand *why* we say the things we do, we are better equipped and informed with the ammunition to say something different. Think about how the world might be if different words were uttered:

Adam might have not blamed Eve; Hitler might have said, "On second thought...." and presidents might just say, "Hey, I lied." Instead, it is our human nature to survive, to be right, and to defend ourselves. This is nearly instinctual in the way we interact with others. Our drive to conquer and control and feed our ego good fried food generally surpasses our innate desire to reach goals, spread joy, and just get along well with others. Gaining a better understanding to why you say the things you say will give you an opportunity to change the way you react. It will not only allow you to see parts of yourself through a different lens, but once revealed, it will make your earlier need to win the ego-war a battle you can finally put behind you.

The ego-centered female is a fairly new phenomenon. It results from females of the past 20 to 30 years struggling for equality; trying to juggle houses, jobs, kids and ex-husbands, often feeling that the world would crumble if they delegated an ounce of the authority they nearly died getting. This is sad and slowly changing, but it is still important to point out that many women are currently suffering from "control-freak syndrome."

Feeling an overwhelming need to control others and the environment around you is a battle you will never win, so you may as well quit trying. The "need to control" in women is not based so much on ego as it is the need to be heard, seen, and felt by those who surround us. Unfortunately, this drive is a result of centuries of subordination, and yet the feeling lingers. Accept right now, before you read another page, that you are only in control of yourself. You do not, *cannot*, control your children, your partner, your employees, or your parents. Everybody on the planet gets the same honor you do: to control one's own thoughts and words. Because control issues are so prevalent (and the number one cause of eating disorders), we will cover them throughout this reading, but now, let's get back to the topic at hand.

While improving our interaction skills so that we can better ourselves, our relationships, and our world is our main intent, understanding of what makes people tick can give you a deeper sense of patience when dealing with them. Once you understand that most people communicate, via ego, you will learn to overlook the "fluff" that currently sends you over the edge in a difficult situation. Not only will that make it easier for you to address the issues that need to be addressed, but you will also be empowered to pursue your goals. Understanding how others think, feel, and *re*act, added to your own sense of self-identification, will help improve how you interact with them.

Chapter Five
THE NEED TO BE RIGHT

NEGATIVE reaction is something we are all guilty of. Regardless of our lot in life, we all want to be right about what we think we know. This drive is already present in children, and probably developed in toddler-hood. We can observe two children in a heated debate that goes something like this: "Did-to," "Did-not," "Did-to!" "Did-not!" Even youngsters are compelled by the need to be right. Historically, this drive has been deeper and stronger in men, to the extent of arm wrestling, fist fighting, and war. However, women feel the need too, only we've managed to masquerade it and, generally speaking, not take it quite as seriously or out onto the street. Still, humans overall seem to be driven by this need to be right.

Carl Rogers, noted psychotherapist, talked about positive regard. Positive regard centers on the fact that we all need warmth, love, and acceptance from other people, particularly those who are most significant, such as our parents. And it's true. We all need to know that we are important and special, if even in our own minds. Perhaps it is our self-imposed lack of confirmation that leaves our egos raging out of control. In essence, we are much like a group of overlooked kindergartners, milling around a room with our finger-painting pictures in hand, looking for someone to tell us what a good job we did.

From youth on, we carry with us this driving need to be recognized, even reckoned with. It is no wonder with this constant need for recognition that we grow into adults who are constantly talking *at* one another instead of *to* one another. Translate this into a typical conversation between a manager and employee.

The manager needs a report re-typed. Her supervisor didn't like some of the verbiage the manager used and asked her to try again. The manager's ego (need to be right) was fairly ruffled, so her attitude is less than enthusiastic when she approaches her assistant for a revision.

"This needs to be done again." the manager says, handing her assistant the paper. In his effort to remain superior, she is not about to tell her assistant that the big boss wanted the work redone. The assistant takes the paper, and instantly assumes she's made a terrible mistake and that her boss is angry with her. In turn, her ego (the need to be right) is consumed with double-checking everything she did on the first draft to see if she can discover the problem. Once she reviews the document and realizes the changes had nothing to do with her work, her attitude will change. Her reaction will be different based upon this new information. There are a few possibilities for how she might feel.

She may be angry that her boss has seemingly changed her mind and wonders why she didn't get it how she wanted it the first time. She might feel indignant that the boss made her feel as if it were her who did something wrong, or she might, depending on the needs of her own ego, feel compelled to make the boss "admit" that the assistant's initial effort was perfect, but that there was another reason the paper needed to be redrafted.

This frequent but unfortunate kind of interaction happens every moment of every day all around the world. It happens at the workplace, in the home, and on the freeway. We are constantly communicating with our egos instead of our heads and our hearts. The need to be right can consume us. So where does it come from and how can we curb its mighty hunger?

Sigmund Freud had some interesting ideas about the ego. Although many of his notions about our secret sexual drives have been discarded and replaced with more modern and realistic theories, he did set the stage for Act One: A Century in Psychoanalysis.

Dr. Freud's exploration of the almighty ego was time well spent. His take on the Super Ego and the Id are still valid in many respects today. What is it about our egos that tell us we need to be right? Essentially, we develop our egos at a very early age. As infants, we develop an "all about me" demeanor, and we never stop nursing it. Emotionally healthy folk have the least depleting "ego-idess." But alas, such a species is all but extinct. Interestingly enough, a low self-esteem can often give the *impression* of an inflated ego, when nothing could be farther from the truth. This probably is true for most of us.

Having an ego is necessary for survival because it can guide us to self-preservation as well as success. It is most effective, however, when couched between common sense and compassion. Besides being a factor for self-identification, the ego can propel us forward in ways that are beneficial to our personal growth.

For example, when you are standing up for something you believe in, assuming it is based on noble intent, your ego is serving you well. Inasmuch, the need to be right can be equally warranted. Take the instance where a parent is persuading a youth that taking drugs is dangerous. Under no circumstances would the parent "give up" his argument for the sake of improved communications. That said, there are times when the need to be right is indeed right. It is instead those times when we are trying to be right simply for the sake of being right that trouble prevails.

In a sales communication workshop given to a group of professional Realtors, this issue of being right comes up often. For example, it is not uncommon for a home-seller to call up the agent and tell her that she thinks the house is priced too low. Often times, the seller was fine with the price the day the house was listed, but since then, has exchanged information with neighbors, friends, and relatives, many of whom came back with a puzzled look, telling her the house was priced too low.

So now the Realtor, a professional who has done her homework, has to contend with a seller who has an idea that is not accurate. Because salespeople, by their very nature, are full of energy and passion, not to mention periodic ego attacks, it is easy to see how this kind of situation can get out of hand. The Realtor knows she is right. Often though, in the heat of the moment, she becomes overwhelmed with "proving" her rightness instead of communicating effectively. This is when deals fall apart, people get fired, and divorce papers are filed. This is the ego making its grand debut.

Being right may be necessary for your success and sometimes your survival. However, *proving* you are right has little significance in the overall world of communications and can seriously impede your important interactions. Furthermore, when you go to any length to prove you are right, simply for the sake of acknowledgement, you are lowering yourself in the eyes of those around you, and that isn't what you want to do.

So why is it so important for us to prove that we are right? Consider the following example:

You are having a discussion with a co-worker about a promotional campaign that is starting in the next week. The ad copy that was being emailed back and forth has mysteriously fallen off the wire and it needs to resurface in order to get the campaign rolling. The conversation goes something like this:

Co-worker: "Last I remember I sent it to you, asking for a few revisions on the closing paragraph."

You: "Yes, and I sent it back to you. I think I only changed a word or two."

Co-worker: "Really? I don't remember getting it back, but I can check."

You: "Yes, please check, I'm sure I did."

Co-worker: "Well, at any rate, I'm sending it out again. If you can get it back to me today, that would be great."

And on the conversation goes on. Even though the main objective is to uncover and/or complete the ad copy, hasn't it turned more into a battle of who is right? Not coincidentally, the corporate culture suffers a great deal of this back and forth who-is- right game of ping-pong. Here's where the ego comes in.

What, if when you were talking on the phone with the co-worker, you were reviewing your backlog of "sent" emails? Kabam! There it is in all its glory—the revision you sent her—just like you said you did. Just like you *knew* you did. How many of us can resist the urge to rub it in her face?

Oh sure, some of us exemplify the true professional and instead of yelling, we whisper. Many of us will fight the childish impulse to shout "Eureka! I found it, I told you! Na, Na, Na." Yet most of us will find a delicate and professionally acceptable way to let the other person know that we were right. We might just forward the older email without saying a word. We've made our statement just the same. We've let the co-worker know that we were right, in order to make our ego shine, while simultaneously offending the other party…and for what? What did we gain from our show(wo)manship? That is the question we must always ask ourselves before our ego takes the reins and proves it knows the answer to all. Now let's look at what compels this need to be right and what the repercussions usually are.

Why was it important that you let your co-worker know you were right? Really think about this. It would be difficult, if not impossible, to learn, grow, and improve your daily interactions with this or any book if you didn't take an active and participative role.

To be a more meaningful and effective communicator you will want to pay attention and apply techniques in both directions. Your concentration will be roughly divided between yourself as speaker and listener, and the other party, as speaker and listener, with the biggest emphasis on you.

That being the case, this approach to improved interactions is two-pronged. First, you must work on yourself by identifying your own communication flaws and striving to improve them. Second, you must realize that the same flaws exist in others. While you can't "fix" anyone else's communication flaws, you can weave your own efforts cautiously over and around in a manner that keeps the currents calm and take you where you are going. You don't always need to be right in front of others.

Chapter Six
LEST WE JUDGE

ANOTHER place the ego often pops up without an invitation is in our judgment of others. As a society we have dedicated so much time to critiquing other people that it has become second nature. It is, however, nearly impossible to conduct meaningful and productive interactions if we're constantly judging everyone we come across.

In *Prospering Women*, Dr. Ruth Ross tells us, "The ego is "I" who we think we are. We created it, and by its very nature, it is limited. When we are in our own ego, we constantly compare and judge ourselves with others." And aint that the truth? Visit any office and listen to the women gossip; flip on day time television; or simply listen to yourself the next time you note how so-and-so needs to drop a few pounds.

Judging others, particularly on petty matters, is something that needs to stop. While men may be just as judgmental on some matters, and it may appear to be more destructive, that is no excuse for the callous and insignificant things we waste our time criticizing. Consider the following: when is the last time you sat in a board room and after the meeting, heard two men whispering by the water cooler, "I can't believe he wore that tie." "I know, and those shoes, what was he thinking?" When we put it that way, it seems silly, yet scores of women at all levels of success participate in such useless, depleting conversations. This raises two issues that must be addressed.

The first issue concerns effective use of time and energy and overall productivity. Judging and gossiping is not a good way to spend your day, a productive way to manifest your goals, or a positive way to contribute to others. The second concerns the "team spirit" of womanhood. These two concerns are reason enough to question yourself next time you partake in needless chitter-chatter gossip toward those who cannot hear what you're saying (and surely wouldn't want to).

When we judge other people, be it male of female, we are sending out a negative kind of energy that will eventually come back to be with us. This is simply the law of cause and effect and it has existed since the beginning of time. To that end, make sure that when you have something less than positive to say about someone else, you won't mind if someone else says the same or worse about you. Additionally, be sure that you would feel comfortable saying whatever negative thing you are saying in front of whoever it is you are saying it about. If not, don't say it.

Sadly, our society has adopted gossiping as just another past time, and unfortunately, we gossip in front of small ears that in turn, learn to say mean things about other people too. Nothing is more disheartening than to hear a child call another child fat, stupid, or ugly, on a playground meant for happier things. Kindness starts where you live. Speaking poorly about others is not kind, no matter how you candy coat it. Moreover, gossiping and mean-spirited comments drive you from your goals and create bad Karma.

Think about saving all of your negative comments and critiques for a whole month, and instead, using that energy and oral effort on things that take you closer to your goals. You will be one hundred footsteps farther on your journey toward success.

People would much rather converse with those who don't gossip and indulge in nasty criticisms of others. Think about the people you have most respected in your lifetime and then consider how much they gossiped. Chances are, it wasn't much. Whole, confident women who love themselves are not constantly driven by the need to criticize other people. Coincidentally, people who experience self-love are quicker to spot the good in others instead of the bad.

Beyond the negative impact judging and critiquing others has on your goals, your time, and your productivity, think about what you are doing to our gender overall. In order for women to elevate themselves universally, they will need to stand on the same platform, open-armed and accepting of one another. You cannot honestly say you love your sisters around the world when you're talking about how tight the receptionist's dress is. Tell the receptionist, but tell her nicely, and only when it's for her own benefit, not yours in disguise. Understand your own drives before you put down the drives of others.

In order to learn more about what drives you, you're going to have to look deep inside the dark places you might ordinarily keep covered. The following exercises have been specifically designed to assist you by challenging you to explore what it is that propels your own need to be right. If you answer these questions honestly (which you should if you expect to excel) many of you will note that your "ego" is merely a protective padding for your insecurities. Identifying what moves you is the first step to every dance. Find out what you need to work on and get busy. Time spent toward improving your communication skills will be one of your wisest investments yet.

Exercise (check "yes" or "no" for each of the following)

1. As a child, I felt loved, honored, and respected
Y_____ N_____

2. In my teen years, I felt that I fit in with an acceptable group of kids
Y_____ N_____

3. I have only been romantically involved with people who respect me
Y_____ N_____

4. I am satisfied with the way I look
Y_____ N_____

5. Sometimes I feel so jealous or threatened by others, I get depressed
Y_____ N_____

6. When I don't win at something I tried very hard at, I become upset
Y_____ N_____

7. When I do win at something I tried very hard at, I feel guilty
Y_____ N_____

8. If someone else gets a promotion, I assume it is because they worked harder or smarter than me- it was my own fault I didn't get it
Y_____ N_____

9. If I am sure I am right about something, I won't stop until I prove it
Y_____N_____

10. When I argue with someone, I become angry if they don't see my point
Y_____N_____

11. I often make comments about people I don't even know
Y_____N_____

12. I often make comments about friends to other friends
Y_____N_____

Now complete the following:

1. If your co-work casually mentions the name of a film she saw, and says the title incorrectly, you gently point out the error. If she disagrees with you, you are most likely to: Let it go_____ See if you can find the correct title somewhere_____

2. In the above scenario, say you see the correct movie title in the newspaper the next day, do you: Clip it out, show your co-worker_____let it go___ mention it_____

3. What if you see the title in the paper the next day, and it turns out your co-worker was right: Clip it out, show your co-worker_____let it go___ mention it_____

4. You are up for a promotion you want very badly. The person you are up against is known as a snake and will try anything to take the job. You just found out she lied about   a project to make herself look better. Do you:
Confront her____tell the boss____ Do nothing about it:_____

5. You and your partner schedule a vacation that you both have waited a long time for. When you finally make your destination, your spouse wants to spend a whole day in a famous museum. You are completely bored by the idea. Do you:
Explain that you've waited too long for this vacation to waste time on something boring_____ Go with your partner, biting your tongue_____ Ask for a compromise_____

The exercise above is not an end in itself. There is no subsequent score sheet. The intent of these exercises is to encourage self-discovery. It is only when we explore our selves deeply that we can begin to understand how and where we fit in with the rest of the world. Think about your answers and what they mean in the overall scheme of things. Many of us need to prove we're right while others of us need to increase our sense of self-worth. There needs to be balance—especially in our interactions with others.

After truly encouraging yourself to explore your ego and the need to be right, think about this: where does it come from? Were you competitive as a child? Were you the youngest, the oldest, or maybe the middle? Dr. Kevin Leman and Randy Carlson tell us in *Unlocking the Secrets of your Childhood Memories,* "As a small child you have certain perceptions of your family atmosphere. You may decide, "This is a place where I need to be in control." Or you may say, "This is a dangerous place that is full of threats and insecurities, I'd better be careful."

It is by no coincidence that many youngsters carry these feelings of insecurity or the need to control into adult life. When we have lived our life this way, as many of us have, it becomes extremely difficult to simply change our way of thinking. As we noted earlier, we've all come across control freaks, some of us surely fit the bill ourselves. The truth is, however, that none of us, no matter how hard we try, can ever be in complete control of anything. Sometimes it rains, cars break down, and people die, and we can't do a thing about any of it.

Managing the need to control everything starts with letting go of the need to run the whole show. Trusting, delegating, and grinding your teeth till your jaw aches are simple steps you can begin with. As you take these quizzes and read this book you might start to see parts of yourself that you've kept comfortably covered up. Now is the time to reveal and reinvent.

The next exercise requires deep and honest thinking. It is by no coincidence that our memories are selective. For example, you might easily remember a disagreement you had two summers ago with your partner (where you prevailed), but your partner can't seem to recall it. It's no coincidence that you were the one who ended up being right in the disagreement. Just as likely, there have probably been many instances when you were incorrect, and someone else was right, but those memories have mysteriously slipped your mind. Now is the chance to recreate some conversations you have already had. These are intended to give you a deeper look at what makes you tick. They will also give you a clearer idea about how being right is really just incidental to the interaction. Real effort and honesty is required on your part in order to reap the biggest self-revealing rewards. This is an opportunity to examine situations you might be in or have been in and to honestly evaluate where you currently stand.

Exercise:

Think about a time in your life when you were in a disagreement with someone and you were right. Now briefly describe the situation:

_____

How did you "prove" you were right?

_____

How did you feel immediately after proving you were right?

_____

How long did that feeling last?

_____

Think about a time in your life when you made a mistake. Now briefly describe the situation:

_____

How did the other person "prove" you were wrong?

_____

How did you feel immediately after?

_____

How long did that feeling last?

_____

When you "win" a disagreement, do you sometimes, in good fun, tease the loser?

_____

When you "lose" a disagreement, how do you feel when the winner teases you?

_____

When you "prove" you are right, does it give you a sense of superiority?

_____

When you are proven wrong, does it give you a sense of failure?

_____

When you know you are correct and someone else is not, are you compelled to prove it?

_____

When someone else thinks they are right, and goes out of their way to prove it, what do you think about that person?

_____

Have you ever yelled or lost your temper at someone because they didn't see your point?

_____

It may be hard to identify parts of yourself you don't find very appealing. We wince when we see parts of ourselves that we perceive as ugly. We need to discard the idea that we must always be picture pretty and perfect. This is hogwash. We are real people intended to sweat and swear and sometimes not feel like washing our hair. It's Okay.

Sometimes it's tough to look at those parts that might suggest we're a little bit insecure and ego-driven. Rest assured—the majority of people you know are insecure and ego-driven. By recognizing and accepting it in yourself, you become empowered to change it.

Furthermore, once you identify it in others, it becomes that much easier to work around.

Knowledge is power.

When reviewing your responses, remember this: there are always exceptions to the rules. If your child is running out in the street to chase a ball, by all means, yell and scream and grab him by the scruff of the neck, dragging him to safety. There are also times when the need to be right, qualifies as a necessity. Say for example you are being audited by the IRS. Now there's an instance when you'll want very much to prove yourself. The point with this practice, like anything else in the world, is that there is a proper place for all things. Here, we are not looking at the extremes, simply acknowledging that they do exist. When we recognize that our interactions with others are often ineffective and ego-driven, we can immediately begin to implement change.

Now we need to dig a bit deeper to see what it is that propels us to act ineffectively. In order to learn effective interaction skills, we need to leave our ego and insecurities outside the situation. In order to do this, we must to identify *why* we feel compelled by the need to be right. If we are simply insecure, as many of us are, we need to work on boasting our self-esteem. If we are overly competitive, perhaps we need to find alternative outlets to enact our competitive nature, such as sports or writing competitions, anything where we can apply our drive to win; just so long as we leave it out of our interactions (if you really need to argue, join a debate team!). Take your time in this next exercise. Read it and think about it before you start writing. This requires a deep and honest look at your internal drives, which is not always so easy (or fun) to spot. Go slow. Be deliberate.

Exercise:
Find the rewards and re-direct them
The need to be right with other people generally satisfies an internal drive. Consider the following scenario and then answer the questions that follow:

Your younger coworker tells you that your budget was a little off, but no problem—she caught it before it was submitted. You know you worked hard on that budget and can't believe you made any errors, especially one that *she* happened to catch. (jot your answers below the questions)

Do you ask to see what the error was?

Do you feel defensive?

Do you feel self-righteous?

Could the coworker just be pulling your chain?

What is it about this situation bothers you?

Does it really make any difference if you made a mistake or not?

If you did make the mistake, aren't you glad it was caught?

If the situation was reversed, and you caught the co-worker's mistake, would you tell her?

Would you wonder, when you told her, why she was acting so defensive?

Would you feel a sense of superiority because she made a mistake?

If you caught the mistake, would you reassure her, telling her everyone makes mistakes (but all the while, feeling relieved that it was her mistake instead of yours)

What is the difference between her making a mistake and you making a mistake?

When she tells you that the mistake was yours, does she seem to be acting superior?

Could you be imagining it?

Do you feel attacked when someone points out an error you make?

How do you think other people feel when you point out errors to them?

Were you reminded of your mistakes as a child? What about as a young adult?

Much of our need to be right is derived from pride. In *The Anger Workbook,* Drs. Les Carter and Frank Minirth explain that unmet needs often result in angry interactions. They also talk about pride, "To understand how pervasive pride is, you will need to set aside stereotyped ideas and stretch your mind to include a very broad spectrum of behaviors. Pride is more than just arrogance or conceit. It is at the core of virtually any unhealthy non-productive emotion or behavior. Specifically, it plays a very influential role in problems with anger." Pride is a key word that is worthy of your consideration. How much of your need to be right is driven by pride? And at closer range, where does it come from? Recognize and address the difference between healthy and unhealthy pride in yourself, and simply notice it in others. It is natural to be proud, for example, because your child scores high on a math test, however, ask yourself, why? Are you proud because the child is a direct reflection of you, so that when he or she accomplishes something, it's as if you made the accomplishment yourself? Or instead, is it a deep love and affection for your offspring and your desire to see him or her achieve greatness? Usually, it's a combination of both, and that's okay; it's human and doesn't hurt anyone.

Pride has its place, so please don't think of it as an unhealthy emotion. It is only when it harms others or drives us in the wrong direction of our goals that it becomes negative. Possessing more awareness about yourself and the role your pride plays in your interactions is an important step you'll need to take. An overactive ego and the need to be right can destroy friendships, marriages, and international relations with rarely any merit. Now that you have had a chance to examine your internal self, you are hopefully a little better informed about the areas you need to be conscientious of when communicating with others. This is an on-going effort. You cannot simply do the exercises and say, "Hurray! I have solved my communication flaws, noted my need to be right, and now all will be well." Unfortunately, things are not that easy.

Yes, the effort you have made thus far says a lot about who you are. It verifies the fact that you recognize the importance of your interaction with others and that you are willing to take responsibility for your share of interaction outcomes in the world. That's more than most ever do. You are already on your way to becoming a brighter light, able to develop genuine and effective interaction skills. From making money, to making babies, to making up, to breaking up; the woman who is in charge of her words is in charge of her world.

In order to more productive you will need to constantly work on those areas you have noted as "weak spots." You will, as luck would have it, run into the very people that seem to challenge your weaknesses more often than you will run into those who validate your effectiveness. Perhaps it is a good measure of and opportunity for personal growth when we are constantly exposed to the exact kinds of people who tend to drive us crazy. At any rate, the first step in effective communications and productive interactions is taking responsibility for your own role in the situation. No placing the blame on someone else for being pushy, wrong, sassy, or slow. Always, always start with yourself.

Understanding and accepting this as a life-long practice is step one. Now let's explore the need to be right in others. Just as you identified in yourself those things that might negatively affect your own reactions, the people you are interacting with will have a collection of their own. Since it's not likely that everyone you run across will have read this book and participated in these exercises, you are shooting somewhat blindly. Still, you may consider yourself officially more equipped than the general population.

The most effective communicators and productive salespeople practice the art of understanding people. While there is no exact science, in spite of an infinite number of books and alleged experts on the subject, understanding people is something everyone should practice. First of all, recognize that human beings cannot be placed into specific categories. Sure, some of us may be quiet, some loud, some friendly, some pushy, some not. The point is that nobody fits neatly inside any shape of box; that's part of being human.

So while people are busy vacillating from yes to no, tomorrow to never, you've got the task of figuring them out. The good news is that the need to be right is fairly easy to spot. If it doesn't come right out and bop you in the head, you'll at least see it standing there. Consider this conversation:

Co-worker: "They're going to paint the offices next week."
You: "This week."
Co-Worker: "I just read the email today, it said next Wednesday."

Now you just happen to be the one who made the appointment with the painters, so you know for sure it's this week, but that's beside the point. Chances are this is a co-worker proudly displaying his need-to-be-right-tail-feathers. Understand that this could just as easily have been you (and probably has been) in the role of the co-worker. When we're right, we're right. This isn't about proving or disproving anything or anyone. Rather, it is about weighing the importance of our rightness against the overall outcome of the interaction.

In the example above, consider the importance of the matter. Say that you are indeed getting your offices painted this week. Say your co-worker is wrong. Understanding the premise behind the need to be right, you will stop and consider the impact. Is there any valid reason you must squelch the co-worker's need to be right?

In other words, will the fact that the painting is going to happen this week opposed to next week really make any life-changing difference to anyone? If it does, then perhaps it will be necessary to prove your point to the need-to-be-right co-worker. If not, let it go.

The truth is that we often find ourselves in scenarios where the other party is overwhelmed with the need to be right. Maybe we're like that too, however, now that we've realized there is usually no direct benefit to it, what's the point?

One client shared a story that serves as a perfect example:

"I walked into the office last month and noticed one of the programmers had the sniffles. I commented something to the effect that maybe she was pushing herself too hard since it seemed that she'd been sick a lot over the past several months. I didn't really mean anything, well, not really. Sure, we're a little competitive, and maybe I was just showing off the fact that I hadn't had a cold all year, but still, it was just a comment. A couple of hours later, I'm on the phone, and here is this programmer, standing at my desk with her timecards in hand! Yeah, she actually went and pulled copies of her time cards so she could show me how many times she had been sick! Me, not having practiced these techniques yet, knew I was right, so together we went through them.

As it turned out, I was right. She had taken 12 sick days before she finally pulled the stack of cards up and said something about it being her mistake and left me sitting there, wondering what in the heck had just happened. I felt right, yes, but more than anything, empty."

This story exemplifies our need to be right. Even the one telling the story tells us how her own need to be right fueled the fire for the programmer's need to be right. The sad part is that the whole communication was pointless. If one of the communicators in the situation above had been the sick programmer's boss, it would present an entirely different set up. But here, we're talking about a pointless interaction, spurred on by an unnecessary comment that should have been dropped or never spoken. Unfortunately, the need to be right took precedence over everything else. It is interaction such as these that you must try to avoid whenever possible. They deplete your energy and are utterly pointless.

Staying with the same situation, imagine yourself in both roles. First, you're the speaker, the one who commented on the frequent illness. This rule is simple: *Think before you speak* firstly, and secondly, *if it might even be remotely related to your ego, don't say it.* This is the best and surest way to keep oneself out of "interaction-interference." You will most often come across this kind of interference when you are dealing with people you feel competitive with. That includes, siblings, co-workers, spouses, friends, enemies, parents, and always those who you feel intimidated or threatened by, if even slightly.

When the roles are reversed and someone makes a comment to you, such as how often you've been out sick, let it go. This is the most challenging, yet easiest way to intercept a comment that drives us crazy. *Learn to let it go.* You might be burning to prove you have been out only two days all year...but, unless this is your boss, what's the point? Do you really thinking proving yourself to your co-worker is going to benefit you in any way whatsoever? If you think for one minute that proving your co-worker wrong is going to bring you any grand prize, go back to page one and start reading again.

Proving someone wrong makes her or him look bad. Can you recall the last time someone made you look bad, and how it felt? Chances are you were in no hurry to take that person to lunch, buy what he was selling, or nominate him for office. When we feed our own ego first, that momentary reward is all we get to eat. When we cast our ego aside, there's a better entrée ahead.

To prove you are right, and moreover, to put any effort at all into *trying* to prove you are right, only solidifies your insecurities for all the world to see, and frankly, is that something you want to show off?

When we let our egos or insecurities overtake our common sense we literally lose control of our selves and the situation at hand. Think about all of the exercises in this chapter. Does "proving" you are right usually change the pattern of the stars and moon, or instead, give you a momentary, otherwise empty, sense of self-righteousness?

In *Communicating at Work,* Drs. Alessandra and Hunsaker warn us how to notice unhealthy communications coming on before they hit, "You need to learn to recognize an emotional reaction coming on by monitoring any increased heartbeat, respiration, or facial flush; physical things that typically happen when you're getting upset about something. When your emotional reaction begins, there is an almost irresistible tendency to interrupt, to butt in, to argue. You lose your train of thought. The first step in controlling this response is to recognize it."

Negative reactions have no place in our communications. They are harmful to our interactions and seldom, if ever, result in anything productive. Reacting negatively ruins your attitude and affects your physical and emotional health by causing stress.

In summary of the Need To Be Right, you'll want to remember the following:

❖ The need to be right is usually always an action of ego insecurity

❖ You don't have to (usually) prove yourself to anyone.

❖ Proving yourself on mute points only lessens your effectiveness.

❖ The best way to deal with others who need to be right is to let them.

❖ Don't intentionally aggravate another person, especially when there is little or nothing at stake, even if you know you are right.

Chapter Seven
DEFENSIVE BEHAVIOR

ANOTHER ego related downfall of communications is defensiveness.
As human beings we are often compelled to defend ourselves against
anything perceived as threatening. As women, we've had to defend
ourselves much more than our male counterpart (often *from* them).
Here though, we are not talking about real threat in the traditional
sense, but rather perceived threat in the self-esteem sense. Ego
defensiveness and the need to be right are almost kissing cousins. A
good way to define and link the two is by considering something we are
all familiar with. Think about when someone else makes a mistake. We
are often the first to notice it, or at least the first to point it out when we
do notice it. If someone misses the ball, we've practically got a running
score in our mind of their entire season of hits and misses. This stems
from our need to be right.

The act of defensiveness then, would best be applied to the
person who is dropping the ball. We know the other guy is keeping
track of our misses and this makes us feel defensive, under scrutiny.
When we're on the defense, we're sure we are being unfairly attacked.
This causes us to put up armor plates and pull out the heavy artillery,
all in an effort to fend off enemy intruders.

In *The Anger Workbook,* the definition of defensive behavior,
"Includes any resistance tactic intended to shield ourselves from
perceived threats. Realistically it is normal to have some defenses
because our world inevitably presents threatening situations. But often,
we overuse our defenses, indicating unresolved fears."

So what are we afraid of? What is it that someone else can say,
often unintentionally, that can send us off the deep end of fear-induced
defensiveness?

Certainly there are times when self-defense is warranted. For
our purpose here though, we are exploring defensive behavior as it
relates to our daily interactions with others and how it holds us back

from getting to our goals, and ruins our relationships. In that realm, it is often more an act of ego-defensive than it is survival.

How many times have you said, or had someone say, "Don't be so defensive?" Being defensive is a natural part of our ego state. It is closely related to the need to be right. Defensive communications can place roadblocks in our interactions and take us farther from our goals. Just as with the need to be right, defensive behavior can be rear its needy head in you, the other person, or both, which creates a real mess. Imagine two people shielding themselves from one another when no one is throwing anything. We shouldn't walk through life that way. Begin by removing your own plate of armor, and then we'll look toward defensiveness in others.

Understanding why and what makes you defensive involves more self-exploration. We all have soft spots or triggers that often evoke a defensive reaction. Perhaps we are feeling guilty or protective about a particular issue when it arises. Other times we are ultra sensitive about a particular subject and tend to react defensively. Many times, however, we act defensive towards others as a result of our own insecurities.

In Dr. Robert M. Bramson's book, *Coping With Difficult People,* he notes that defensive behavior, of a non-physical nature is, "Most frequently psychological, and the deepest wounds we get from it, is our motivation and feelings of self-worth."

It becomes evident then, that in order to become more productive in our interactions, we need to learn how to eliminate unnecessary, defensive behavior. The only way to do this effectively is by examining what kinds of things make us feel as if we're being attacked.

It is time again to participate in an exercise. Here we will dig deeper into your personal defense triggers by identifying and attempting to work through them.

Exercise:

1.   You draw a map up so that a co-worker can meet you for a business meeting the next day. When he arrives, he is flustered and attributes it to the poor directions you provided. You realize, after looking at it, you made a mistake. How do you feel?_____Are you able to just let it go, or do you dwell on it? Worse yet, do you find something negative about your co-worker to justify your own error? Was being defensive helpful to resolving the issue? Was there really an issue to deal with?

2.   Your boss gives you a review and explains he would like to see a dramatic improvement in your organizational skills. What is the first, defensive reaction you feel?_____ Is feeling defensive in this case going to help resolve the issue?

3.   Your partner blows up over something that you think is seemingly small, and then tells you that you never think of anyone but yourself. What physical feelings to you notice?_____What is the first emotional feeling that this situation presents?_____Is feeling defensive bringing you closer to resolving the issue?

Which of the following words come to mind when thinking about the cases above:

Threatened
Insulted
Embarrassed
Stupid
Attacked
Wronged
Accused
Humiliated

Abused
Foolish
Mistaken
Corrected

Now name the person(s) or situation(s) from your past that evoked similar feelings as the words from the word list you selected above. Think back and try and recapture the feeling, even if it is uncomfortable to do:

_____

_____

_____

_____

Consider what occurrences from your past might set off triggers even now and then think about ways of letting them go.

Hopefully, these exercises have given you enough ideas about how you might react defensively and how you might reinvent those feelings. A good rule of thumb for recognizing when you might react defensively is whenever you describe the situation as "feeling attacked." When we feel like we're being attacked, we run for cover. We defend our self, our actions, and our honor. We don't see, at that particular point, how negative this kind of reaction appears to others, particularly when no harm was intended. Yes, there are times when someone might indeed be intentionally offensive in their tone or with their words, but even then, is reacting defensively going to get the interaction back on track?

Reacting defensively is harder to deal with than the need to be right because while the need to be right fills us with a false sense of superiority, defensiveness leaves us feeling trampled and helpless. Feeling helpless continues to be an unwelcome guest for most of us. When we feel helpless, it is like being trapped in a cage; we will say or do anything to escape, hardly giving a second thought to our captor. Think about how harmful this might be in the case where our captor isn't really a captor at all.

The key to dealing with defensive reactions in your self is an ancient yet simple remedy: *don't take it personal.* Presumably, you have taken the exercises thus far and are feeling a little bit more knowledgeable about your personal defensive reaction triggers. Perhaps more exploration is warranted. At any rate, once you are at that point of self-awareness, the rest can consist of simply doing as the ducks do: let it roll right off your back.

Don't Take it Personally

This doesn't mean that there are not times when telling the other person you feel attacked or trampled is not in order; we all have that right. It does mean, however, that you understand the fact that no one else really has the power to make you feel any emotion you're not already allowing yourself to feel, regardless of the words they say.

Defensive reaction is more challenging to overcome than the need to be right. When we feel the need to be right, we may experience a flash of excitement or a need to jump up and announce the truth, yet these are emotions we can, with a bit of effort, learn to control. We can bite our tongue and forget about it, secure enough that we can let it slide. When we feel offended though, it's not always so easy to bite our tongue or let it slide.

Feeling offended often involves much more vulnerability than the simple need to be right. Here, the ego is at the polar opposite of cocky self-assuredness. When we feel attacked our feelings get hurt and that is often more difficult to overlook. Learning not to take things personally is the first and foremost step in resolving the issue. Once we accomplish this, we begin to realize that not everything everyone says to us is gospel, or said with the intent to harm. Learning to let things slide is an enormous element in developing more productive interaction skills. In essence, we give away tremendous amounts of time and energy over insignificant comments that other people make. When we do that, we give away our power. Become aware of the kinds of triggers that cause you to feel defensive and learn to overcome them.

Moreover, it's important to recognize what kinds of comments make other people feel defensive.

So what about when we say something to someone else and he or she feels personally offended? How often have you uttered seemingly innocent words and stood by surprised to see those words transformed an otherwise calm communication into a bona fide screaming match? Sometimes we don't even know what it is we said that set the room on fire.

The problem with a defensive reaction is this: it would be literally impossible to explore and understand the nuances, soft spots, childhood traumas, and communication styles of every single person we are ever going to interact with. Of course, the caveat is that you should take special steps to be as aware of these elements in those you interact with intimately and infinitely as much as humanly possible. This, of course, is not reasonable in and with our most common connections; co-workers, supervisors, neighbors, acquaintances, and the guy who changes the oil in our car. Even when we are aware of words that trigger defensiveness in others, we still sometimes use them, maybe intentionally, hopefully not. The point is that we cannot be responsible for the emotional reactions of other people, but we *can* control our words and use them to the best of our ability.

When you do find yourself in an interaction where you have struck a sensitive chord, all you can do is apologize and move on. There is little sense in saying,"Don't be so defensive," as that only tends to intensify the problem (does it help when someone says that to you?). It hardly seems necessary to remind you that you should always avoid communications that you already know, through intuition or experience, will intentionally make the other person feel defensive. To do otherwise is not only ineffective, it is cruel and takes you miles farther in the wrong direction of your intent to do and be well in the world.

There are some situations where, regardless of what you say, the other person is going to react defensively. For example, think about firing someone. This is easily one of the most dramatic blows to a person's self-esteem. Careful communications can soften the blow, while thoughtless ones can worsen it.

Consider this scenario: Phil is a very nice guy, only he spends too much time socializing. So much time in fact, that many employees have complained about him, and as a result, productivity has fallen. You are his boss and have been informed by higher ups that his talkativeness is costing the company money and he must be terminated at once.

Regardless of how this is handled, Phil is getting fired just the same, right? Well, yes and no. The way that you, as Phil's boss, handle the termination, can greatly impact Phil's overall reaction. Sure, initially he will feel bad; anyone does when they get fired. By handling it effectively though, Phil will be much less defensive in how he reacts, both immediately and in the long run.

The thoughtless communicator might say:

"I have to fire you Phil, you're just too much of a distraction." This would obviously leave Phil feeling very defensive and emotionally wounded. Consider an alternative approach:

"Phil, you're a great guy. You're very social and friendly and everybody likes you, only, this isn't a place where overly social people tend to do very well. It seems to cause the other workers too much of a distraction, and that's a problem. Perhaps you should consider a position that is more people-oriented. I'm sorry Phil, but we're going to have to let you go. We'd be happy to give you a good recommendation, and we wish you all the best."

Either way, Phil got fired. But if you were Phil, which termination would you feel better about? The second one is clearly the lesser of two evils. With the second approach, Phil might feel bad at first, but chances are he'll bounce back a lot quicker than he would by simply learning that he's out of a job. At least in the second example he has learned what not to do, or perhaps even what he does well, and he can proceed from there.

There are no perfect canned patterns of speech that we can pull out of our magic hats to make sure we say the right thing every time. However, recognizing the roles our ego plays helps us in two undeniable ways.

First, by identifying our own triggers and weak spots, we can greatly reduce our negative reactions to others. It takes time and self-acceptance to improve the way we react to the words that other people say. As you become more patient with yourself and others you will note improved reception; people seem more agreeable, less argumentative and nicer to be around. Even the smallest effort to interact beyond your ego will make a marked difference.

Secondly, when we realize that the people we talk to are just as likely to feel the need to be right and feel wounded and defensive, we are better able to act accordingly. We can avoid terms and tones that might be negatively construed. At first, we might have to bite our tongue and swallow the blood. Eventually though, we learn to recognize that the triggers coming from others are most often their own egos and insecurities at work. Knowing this makes it easier to let go and walk around. Even the first few side steps can make a difference. When people don't feel us reacting to their egos, they tend to feel more comfortable setting them aside; putting down the armor and letting go the ammunition.

We've looked at the underbelly of bad communications by understanding that we have two choices in working with other people. We can be productive or not. Reacting negatively, that is, wearing our egos and insecurities like a new silk skirt, leaves us empty and alone. It hurts our relationships and stymies our effective communications. We can't confidently capture our goals or contribute to the rest of the world if we're busy babying our ego. Learn to say it nice, or learn to let it go.

WHEN YOUR WORDS FAIL YOU

Before we can understand the Effective Response Theory, we must first be able to identify what is *not* effective, what doesn't work. This goes a little bit beyond the basic ego/insecurity stuff we covered in the last chapter. The "gremlins" of ineffective communications are: not listening, yelling, and over reacting. In addition to reviewing how these look in real life, we're going to explore the results that these negative interactions have on our physical and emotional well-being.

Not listening is a communication flaw we are all well aware of. How many times have you been in conversation with someone else and missed half of what she said because you were so busy preparing your response? Consider the following conversation:

> **Carol:** *How was your weekend?*
> **Sue:** *Great! I went up in my first hot air balloon.*
> **Carol:** *Cool. I remember my first ride. We drank champagne and ended up coasting over the hills of Napa.*
> **Sue**: *Oh.*

This example appears innocent enough, however, examine the missing factor. Carol failed to acknowledge Sue's adventure. She could have inquired more about the experience; given Sue a chance to elaborate on her adventure. What Carol did is something many of us tend to do and something we recognize much quicker in others. Unfortunately, we tend to overlook this fault in ourselves. The outcome of this kind of interaction is that the person that was not adequately listened to, feels ignored, not important, invisible. Often this lack of listening is a result of our attempt to "out do" someone else's adventure or story.

How can we communicate effectively if we make the other person feel bad? Is making someone else feeling like less in any way productive? Moreover, consider the relationship at hand. If this is a prospective client, a child, or an employee, do you really think that making the person feel less than spectacular about her/his self is going to foster any kind of positive motivation?

People need to be heard. It's very human to need to know that someone has heard what you said and then subsequently acknowledged it. Think it over. That is why the infamous cold shoulder routine we discussed earlier has remained the number one overused and abused conflict strategy throughout the ages. It's petty and immature and drives people crazy. We all want validation that what we have to say is worth listening to.

Not listening during emotionally intense interactions can be very destructive. When we are not listening to what the other person says in a conflicting communication, we are setting ourselves up for failure. Replying to something someone says before fully listening and acknowledging the words is also a mistake. Not listening could very well be the number one complaint in marriages and customer and employee dissatisfaction. Even when people are verbally acknowledged, it may not be enough. People need to know that they are being listened to on all levels. We need to take time to *hear* what is being said.

It's been estimated before that nearly 90% of all medical visits are essentially for reassurance. People go to the doctor or emergency room because they need someone to tell them everything will be all right. They need someone to kiss their "owies" and make them feel better. This is the same reason people spend oodles of money on mental health.

It is not to say that therapy and counseling are without merit, quite the contrary, an infinite number of individuals have turned their lives around with the positive impact of therapeutic support. It is, however, to say that people who go to therapy are really, at a basic level, paying someone to hear them. To listen to what someone has to say without placing judgment is a multi-billion dollar industry. We all need to be heard, and when you take the time to listen to those who are trying to talk, you will move mountains with your silence.

Right along side not listening is "jumping the gun." Jumping the gun is very similar to not listening, only more aggressive. When you jump the gun, you tend to think you know what the other person is going to say before they say it, and then react as if they had already said it. This can obviously present enormous problems in heated discussions and can be quite annoying in everyday conversations.

Wife: *The telephone company called today and said....*

Husband: *I told you that bill wasn't paid. Don't you ever listen to me?*

Wife: *...they received double payment and were issuing us a credit.*

Husband: *Oh. Sorry.* (that is, if she even gets a sorry out of him!)

Do you see how in this conversation the husband jumped the gun? How do you suppose this made his wife feel? What impact might it have on their relationship? Imagine if it were instead, a professional interaction. While we tend to blow off more steam in our personal life with those we feel closest to (which makes less sense than anything), there are people who don't think twice about snapping back or jumping the gun in a professional setting. Not only does this destroy team spirit and working relationships, it also causes people to be much less likely to voluntarily present information and ideas for fear of being interrupted or overlooked. This is destructive for any business as well as the individual interactions of those involved.

Jumping the gun is never a productive way to communicate and is often the catalyst for ruined relationships. People feel rejected when other people pounce on them. Rejected and attacked and fed up with the world. People who live together, especially couples, as well as parents toward their children, tend to be the quickest at reacting before the other person finishes. Bite your tongue until it bleeds if you need to, but always remember to let the other person have a say. It will be appreciated, and it will improve the outcome of the interaction dramatically.

Listening is important. By simply listening to what the people around you say you will endear yourself to others. People are practically accustomed to being interrupted and ignored. Start listening fully with all of your attention and notice how fast you become the most popular person in the office, the home, or any other place you might be. It is by no coincidence that when you are a good listener people tend to think you're wiser, friendlier and easier to talk to than most.

It's true. If you were to observe any group of various conversations, people who listened well to others would easily be voted the best conversationalists, even if they didn't speak at all! People tend to gravitate toward people who will listen to them. Being heard is our society's way of saying, "you are acceptable." If someone is willing to listen to you, you must have something good to say.

While not listening is certainly one way to ensure poor communications, nothing gets you there quicker than being a yeller.

People who lose their cool and raise their voices fall off party lists rather quickly. Loud voices represent anger, and people don't like to be subject to, or victim of, anyone's screaming frenzy.

Nobody likes to be yelled at. It doesn't matter if we're talking about a child, a dog, an employee or a spouse. Nobody likes to be yelled at. As a matter of fact, people hate it. Unfortunately, we live in a high-stress society where we're all moving at warp speed to accomplish unrealistic goals. When things get in our way, we often react ferociously. Fortunately, there is a very simple way to avoid this behavior in your self.

In *Lions Don't Need To Roar,* Debra Benton tells us, "If you control your actions, you can control your effect to control you career." She goes on to say that this practice is critical in our interactions with others. Put another way, it's vital that you learn to harness your emotional outbursts. There is not now, nor will there ever be, a time when yelling is an effective means to an end.

Think back to a time when you were in a department store, bank, or restaurant and someone got upset and began to yell at the clerk. Maybe you were at the phone company billing-desk— people tend to lose their cool quickly where money is concerned. In this scenario, someone became obviously enraged and started yelling at someone behind a counter who was trying very hard to keep his or her cool.

Remember how you held your head down? You were probably rolling your eyes at the other people in line, thinking how glad you are that *you* never act like that. The person who was yelling was turning red and demanding action of some sort or another. The poor clerk looked brow beaten half to death, and finally was rescued by the manager, who managed to calm down the angry customer.

Nearly all of us have witnessed this situation, or one fairly similar. Generally speaking, people will yell not only when they feel they've been wronged, but also when they feel somehow equal to or superior to the person they are yelling at. This is why you might see an employee tolerating an angry boss, or a child bowing his head in fear at the sound of a yelling parent; we tend to cower down to those who have some kind of perceived power over us. Unfortunately, this has prevailed for far too along among women and the men who over power them. It's not okay for someone to yell at you just because they're bigger.

In the scene above, how was the manager able to calm the customer who was yelling? Chances are that the person yelling has finally figured out what a fool he's made of himself. Once the manager enters the scene, calmly and quietly and listening, the person calms down too. The moral of the story is that yelling will never ever take you closer to your goal, but listening always will.

This is not brain surgery or advanced calculus. These are simply rules that we all know but let fall through the cracks when they don't suit our needs. Or, maybe we don't know the rules because our own role models forgot to teach them to us. It does not take an aerodynamic engineer to teach you that you shouldn't yell at the Kmart clerk or that you should listen to your third grader's side of the story before you blow a gasket. However, it is the simple rules of the road that we often tend to overlook. Unfortunately, a seemingly small mistake, like speeding on the street, can cause many head-on collisions.

While you cannot control another person's reaction or temper, you can always control your own. As far as contending with people who yell at you, the best advice is to walk away. Hang up the phone, go in the house or leave the scene. No one has the right to verbally abuse you, and yelling in your face is verbal abuse. If it is a relationship worth keeping, you can resume the conversation when the other person has calmed down. It is time for women to stake their claim in physical equality. Just because somebody is bigger or stronger or has a deeper voice does not give him the right to overpower your being. Grab your hat, a bat, or the car keys and leave well enough alone. Never acquiesce to something if and when you can possibly help it. People can only treat you badly if you allow it.

This applies to customers as well. Keeping customers happy is clearly a priority, but that does not give them a license to yell at you. You will find, in most cases, that if you learn to control your own anger, other people will follow suit. When this is not true, take care of yourself in whatever way you can and refuse to prolong the battle.

The easiest way to keep your cool in times of interaction-trouble is to ask yourself a very simple question: *What will this change?* In any given situation, will yelling serve to improve the interaction? Chances are invariably not. Will yelling make you easier to communicate with? Again, the answer is no. Furthermore, consider the fact that you cannot "unyell" at someone. Once you have yelled, you might be able to apologize afterward, however, there is nothing you can do to change the fact that you yelled in the first place. No one in all the history of the world has ever unyelled.

If you are at a department store trying to return a product that was broken when you bought it and the clerk is giving you a hard time, your natural reaction is to yell; to lose your cool, raise your voice, and maybe even make a scene. Some of us yell softer than others, but we all get mad at people who stand behind counters at one time or another. You have to ask yourself the qualifying question: will getting mad help the situation? Will it make the interaction run smoother? Will you be a better communicator because you yelled at the person behind the counter or on the other end of the telephone?

The answer is nearly always an unequivocal no. An angry response or attack in our communications will not promote productive interactions. Yelling will not inspire people to want to support you. It will only give them a bad feeling in the pit of their stomach and make them want to yell back (even if they don't or can't).

In summary, the two things you can do that will have the biggest negative impact on your communications is to not listen and to yell, or otherwise lose your cool. If you interrupt other people when they are speaking, fail to acknowledge what they have said, ignore their words, reply rudely or in anger, you have most assuredly broken the golden rules of human interaction. Furthermore, you have added to the negativity of the world. It is our mission to maximize our power and potential by bringing more positive energy to the planet, not less.

Let's close the subject on ineffective communications by taking a closer look at how non-productive communications in everyday settings affect our lives. The purpose here is to illustrate that negative reactions can really wreck your world. In addition to ruining the day, non-productive communications can negatively impact the relationships you've worked hard to build, the goals you've set out to reach, and the health you hope to maintain. We will explore how this happens through two examples, each followed by an analysis that's easy to understand.

You and a co-worker have been charged with completing a very important budget that will be presented to the Board of Directors in two days. After completing your portion of the project, your co-worker tells you to go home, she will finish her part and it will be waiting for you when you arrive in the morning.

Anxious, you get to work early only to find the co-worker didn't work on the report at all. She walks in twenty-minutes later, while you've been chomping at the bit. Your anger is easy to spot and you practically jump at her when she walks in the door.

> *"Why isn't this done?"* you demand.
> *"Sorry, something came up."*
> *"Something came up? Do you know how important this is?"*
> *"I said I was sorry, we'll have to catch up now."*
> *"Sorry isn't good enough when my promotion is on the line."*

STOP

Now let's ask and answer the following key communication/ interaction questions:

1. Was this communication productive?
2. Did this interaction positively affect the relationship?
3. What physical implications did this communication have?
4.

Starting with number one. No, the communication was not productive. In this case, productive would have meant that the budget was going to get completed under the best conditions possible. The way this is looking, that's not going to happen. A productive communication is one that brings you closer to your goal, but never farther away.

Number two. No, the interaction did not have any positive affect on the relationship between you and your co-worker. If anything, you feel like you've carried more of the burden and that you cannot communicate with or trust your co-worker for future projects. By not probing deeper with fact-finding questions (which we will discuss in section two), you only reacted to the situation in a way that left your co-worker feeling defensive and disagreeable.

Number three. This is the one we seldom stop and think about. The interaction above did, however, have an implication on your health. Unless you are a Zen Master, this kind of situation would inevitably stress you out. When you feel a substantial degree of stress that tends to last for more than just a few minutes, there are physical ramifications. Your body reacts to stress by assuming the flight or fight syndrome, causing your heart rate to increase and other bodily functions to speed up when they're not supposed to.

If we're always exposing ourselves to tremendous amounts of stress, our health will most certainly be affected. There is no way around it. If you can't control the stress in your life, expect to pay the price, eventually. One of the main contentions of this book is to bring to light that the greatest degree of our daily stress is directly related to negative interactions with others, and that if we can learn to improve our interactions with others, we can reduce the amount of stress we experience. As a result, we'll not only get closer to our goals in life, but we'll be healthier too!

In the example above, the physical implications are easy to spot. First of all, you would feel anxiety because the budget is not complete and your promotion depends upon it. That would cause anyone to feel a great deal of stress. Of course, it does not help matters that your verbal interaction with the co-worker did not take you closer to the goal of completing the budget, but seemingly farther away. Next, the wedge in your relationship has been planted. Whether or not you were friends to begin with doesn't much matter; it doesn't take a scientific study to show us that when we harbor bad feelings for others, and they for us, we are emotionally affected.

It should be easy to see then how our interactions impact our physical and emotional well-being. Remember, stress cannot only make us feel bad, but more and more medical research is proving that stress can be directly related to a myriad of degenerative diseases. Our interactions with others are not supposed to make us sick.

Let's look at another example, this time one that might occur on the home front. Personal scenarios are often more volatile for a number of reasons. First of all, when you are dealing with someone personally, you don't have the professional demeanor you always feel compelled to keep up at work. In other words, at the office, we will mind our manners at any expense, while with a partner, offspring, or department store clerk, we tend to let it all come pouring out. Another reason personal interactions are more delicate is because they are often more important to us so we tend to be more sensitive to their content. We are more emotionally invested, involved and charged. When you become enraged with a co-worker, you can go home, thankful that you only have to tolerate him on a limited basis. When it's your life-partner, however, there is no anticipated escape (hopefully) and this is someone that you presumably are spending a fair amount of social and personal time with; time that is meant to be pleasurable, not laborious.

Perhaps this is why it's so important to practice our communication skills at home even more than we do at work. Most people tend to be consumed with corporate communications. Yes, understanding how to interact at the office can dramatically improve your chances for professional growth and personal contentment. However, never underestimate the power of personal relationships and how growing in these areas can have tremendous and positive affects on the rest of your world. Best selling author Thomas Stanley, Ph.D., tells us in *The Millionaire Mind,* that the vast majority of self-made millionaires he worked with and interviewed all had happy stable home lives. Family was frequently the first priority and most of the millionaires had been married to the same spouse forever.

You would be hard pressed to have a miserable home life and come to work productive and approachable each day. You wear your world on your sleeve whether you think you do or not. Master the art of personal interactions and office talk will be a breeze.

Now let's look at a home-based interaction. In this example, your teenage daughter has missed curfew. You waited up for two hours on a busy weeknight only to find her sneaking in at midnight. You practically attack her in the hallway.

> *"Where were you?"*
> *"Sorry Mom."*
> *"Sorry doesn't cut it, I was worried sick!"*
> *"Well Cindy had a....."*
> *"I don't care what Cindy had, you are grounded Missy, don't even think about going out on a weeknight again."*
> *"But Mom..."*
> *"But nothing...go to bed."*

When you read this it might appear exaggerated, or as if the mother was overly harsh. Or, it might seem to you like she was completely justified, particularly if you have a teenage daughter of your own. In reality though, this happens to be quite a typical, yet unacceptable, scenario. As parents, we don't always relinquish control of our children and that often carries over into our interactions. Today, more than ever, it is vital that we develop strong and open communications with our children. Sending them away without giving them a chance to speak is child rearing from another century. Today, we can't operate our relationships like that and expect to develop healthy happy families.

In the example above, you answer the questions.

1. Was it productive?
2. Did it positively impact the relationship?
3. What physical implications did it have?

Hopefully, you can easily identify that the Mother-daughter interaction was not productive (she didn't address the issue or hear what the daughter had to say), didn't have a positive impact on the relationship, and certainly caused stress and anxiety (probably for both of them).

In conclusion, *ineffective* communications are essentially *negative* reactions. When we react negatively, we bring all our bad baggage into the interaction and nothing worthwhile seems to get accomplished. Even if we do achieve our goal, if it is done through ineffective communications, we'll inevitably suffer stress and ill feelings for ourselves and in others.

Our egos, insecurities, and impatience account for just about all of our communication flaws. Generally speaking, the ego/insecurity factor propels us to "prove" our rightness or fend off communications that are interpreted as attacks. Our impatience causes us to lose our cool and bring hostility into interactions that we would be better off without.

Most of our ego-reaction stems from our childhood and the things that we grew up believing about ourselves.

Doctor Susan Vaughan, in her book, *Half Empty Half Full*, tells us, "For every child who emerges from childhood having essentially learned to tame the beasts of anger, anxiety, and sadness, and having been equipped with representations of him self and others in relationships that are infused with positive emotions, there is another less unfortunate child. His early life experiences have left him with cognitive-affective structures in which powerful negative feeling states like shame, anger, guilt, contempt, and loneliness play a central role."

These structures that form in youth, positive or negative, will eventually surface in relationships with others. It becomes easy to see that the things we learned to believe about ourselves when we were young are directly related to our style of interacting as "big people," when we are supposedly all grown up.

It is by no coincidence that negative interactions seem contagious. Beyond our own need to be right and act defensively, when we see other people react negatively, it is easy to follow suit. Roland Neumann, Ph.D., conducted a study that demonstrated people who listened to a sad speech, became sad and when they listened to an upbeat speech, became happy. This explains why you can start out the day feeling robust and sophisticated, spend a few hours with your mother, and feel like the whole world stinks.

Moods, outlooks, and attitudes have an inordinate affect on us. That means you need to protect yourself from surrounding negativity, and ensure that you're sending out only the good stuff.

Another study by psychologist David G. Myers noted that when we communicate with others we mimic their facial expressions and speech rhythms. The study indicated that in spending as little as twenty minutes with someone who is angry or depressed causes us to assume similar emotions.

These studies indicate some pretty powerful ideas. Namely, that if you communicate with someone who becomes reactive, it's entirely possible that you too, perhaps unconsciously, will act the same. You have to pay attention to what you say before it comes out of your mouth. Learn to monitor yourself, particularly in situations that are potentially sensitive or volatile. Do not allow someone else's negative reaction to cause the same in you. People with a healthy outlook on life communicate effectively; people that communicate effectively can acquire a healthy outlook on life.

Virtually all modes of miscommunications that end in emotionally heated discussions do so because we feel, on some level, threatened. When we feel good about ourselves, we tend to feel good about other people. It becomes clear that working on our own issues of insecurity, low self-esteem, and anger control become paramount factors toward improving our interaction skills. This includes mood control as well. It is not fair that we come home and yell at our children because we were stuck in the rush-hour traffic. This is nothing short of a lack of self-control and responsibility on our part, and all too common in many households and corporate offices across the country.

Start now by paying attention to the way you talk to others. Notice when you feel compelled to be grumpy, snap back, prove your point or give someone the cold shoulder, what's going on inside your head. Watch your mood and watch your mouth; keep in control of your communications and you control your world.

The exercises provided up until this point have been especially designed to help you get a better grasp on those communication flaws that stand between you and happy healthy interactions. If you find that you are lacking in a specific area, please spend extra time and additional effort into working through this weakness. You will be pleasantly and productively surprised when you learn the important role your communication skills play in your own life, when you use them to your advantage.

Now that have explored what not to do, let's address the heart of the matter, the Effective Response Theory.

Before you go on, why not take a few moments and jot down on a pad of paper or in a journal some things that you have learned, realized, or recognized about yourself and your own interactions. Remember, self-discovery is key in the learning process and absolutely essential in reaching our goals.

Chapter Eight
EFFECTIVELY YOURS
(The Effective Response Theory)

THE Effective Response Theory takes its cues by combining the discipline of psychology and communications theory. The best of both worlds: how we feel and what we say. Here we can temper compassion with common sense, kindness with keeping our eye on the carrot. Here we can learn to have it all by the words we use and the way we use them.

Beyond that, the premise was built on the frustration of watching women earn MBA's, but not be able to speak effectively to co-workers, or seeing mothers unable to communicate with their own children, or worse still, seeing us all use our words as weapons instead of the useful tools they were intended to be.

This Theory is so simple to follow that it could be taught to; school-aged children, CEOs, students in anger management classes, parents, teachers, and corporate workers across the country. It is simple because it is no more than learning to talk nicely. Learning to listen. Learning to think about how the other person feels and then speaking accordingly.

After studying the ego-response, as outlined in the first section of this book, it became clear that the initial step to improved interactions starts within each of us. The adage is true: *you can only control yourself,* and this is where we shall start.

Once we've identified what propels us forward, what our individual triggers are, we are better equipped to handle them. Once we understand why we say the things we do, or feel a certain way when someone says something that doesn't sit quite right with us, we become more powerful communicators, more intuitive in our interactions. Furthermore, by understanding the ideas set forth in section one, we are more clear as to how ego, insecurity and anger play a role in the communication efforts of others. So, while we can't necessarily change the way other people communicate, we can at least begin to understand that bad behavior in others is out of our control. We don't take it as personally as we might have before. A quote by Ethel Barrett says, "We would worry less about what others think of us if we realized how seldom they do." And it is true. We worry, beginning in our conscientious youth, that all eyes are on us, when usually it's just not true. We need to realize that just as we are consumed with our self, everyone else is equally consumed with his or her own life. People don't spend nearly the time thinking and talking about us as we might imagine.

Accepting human nature and becoming self-aware is the foundation for a better way to get along. When we communicate from our hearts and heads instead of our ego and insecurity, we increase our productivity, feel better physically and emotionally, and allow ourselves to be the kind of women other people like to support and assist. We become the change we want to see in the world.

The Effective Response Theory is comprised of several parts. The first relates to understanding our audience, our attitudes and expectations, and ethical interactions. The real crux of the theory develops from that point on. Primarily, Effective Response Theory (ERT) consists of the following steps:

- ➢ Identify Goals
- ➢ Step Outside
- ➢ Walk in Their Shoes
- ➢ Ask/Listen
- ➢ Respond Effectively

Your communication skills will rate par excellent once you begin to incorporate these strategies in the various interactions that you have. The steps are very simple, but the idea behind them is that you learn to apply them simultaneously. This is what we will work on.

While each step matters independent of the others, it won't work as well if you only perfect one area and overlook the rest. The key is to understand the sequence of steps and then apply them accordingly. The exercises toward the end of the book have been specifically designed to help you learn to streamline the steps so that they become intentionally integrated. With practice, anyone can be proficient.

And, there is always time for practice. In reality, we have the rest of our speaking, listening lives to communicate. Wouldn't we be better off to at least try and improve the way we do it? This application will give you a foundation that you can build upon, until interacting with others becomes one of the biggest joys of your life, as it should be.

This section of the book will take you by the hand and demonstrate how easy it is to become the most effective communicator in the office, the home, or anywhere. Additionally, when you take the time and make the effort to improve yourself, others around you cannot help but be changed, improved. Your interaction skills expand and so do your relationships, health and overall productivity. Think of the possibilities.

LAYING THE GROUNDWORK

BEFORE we dive head first into Effective Response Theory (ERT), it's important that we lay the groundwork. In the first section we looked at what gets in the way of effective communications, now let's look at what works, starting with the foundational rules. In order to be effective, we need to understand the audience, address our own attitude, and remember the importance of honesty and ethical behavior.

For our definition, your audience is the person or people you are talking to. For these purposes, we're really referring to one other person, but don't think for a minute that these ideas and techniques won't work for communicators of all contexts—they will. It doesn't matter if you're talking to the UPS clerk, a co-worker, your partner, or the next-door neighbor; you need to understand your audience. This doesn't mean you need to psychoanalyze everyone you meet. It merely means that, just as you have a reason to communicate with them, they have one for communicating with you, and it is helpful to know what that reason is.

The sooner you can identify the motivation, the better off you are. If we're talking about a store clerk, it's easy to see that the reason he is there is because he's getting paid to be there. Besides that simple example, it's not always so easy to see what drives people, or what it is they need from us. People often have hidden agendas and it would do you well to try to see beyond the surface of what is being said. It's not really all that difficult to read people. Simply pay attention to eye contact, body language and gestures, and you'll have a pretty good idea of whose shooting from the hip and who is not. Generally speaking there are two basic motivations that psychologists refer to: internal and external.

External drives induce results such as recognition, awards, rewards, and praise. Internal drives are more related to our own sense of self-worth and goal-setting challenges. In other words, if a student participated in an essay-writing contest and won, the external drive would be the $50 prize and recognition from her instructors and peers. The internal drive would be from her sense of self-satisfaction that he met the goal successfully. Generally speaking, we are propelled farther by internal goals, as many athletes will attest to. Also generally speaking, men tend to be more self-driven and women historically are more driven in the art of helping others. Again, balance is key.

This doesn't mean that you should chuck the charity work and climb some corporate ladder (unless that's what you want to do), what it does mean is that you should learn to apply as much effort and passion into your own goals as you do the goals of your partner, your children, your "group."

When we strike balance in giving and taking, we find our rewards are many. There is nothing more gratifying (or universally compensated) than being of service to others. However, there is also a great deal of honor in taking care of your self. When you work on your more dreams you are creating even more opportunity to serve others, that's just the way it works. So back to motivation.

Breaking your own record or achieving your own goal is somehow a more powerful incentive than a trophy and a smile. Don't misunderstand, however, having both internal and external motivators is the most effective of all. Receiving accolades could arguably be intrinsic or extrinsic depending on which psychologist you might be talking to. The point is to recognize that next to winning the lottery, one of the best rewards in life is when people prove to themselves and others that they are valuable and successful.

How this pertains to *your* interactions is best displayed with an example.

If you have a report that is vital to finish and you know it's time for your assistant to leave for the day, short of ineffectively demanding her to stay, ask yourself what would motivate her. Here is where you look to internal and external drives. If she is primarily motivated by external drives, then to offer her something in the way of incentive or reward could work. For instance, offer to take her to a nice lunch the next day, or tell her she can come in late, or leave early the next day. People that are motivated by external rewards often require something tangible that they can hold in their hand.

More often than not though, people are motivated by internal rewards. In this case, letting your assistant know how vital she is to the success of the project and making sure she gets ample credit will take you far with this favor, as well as the next one. People who are internally driven are seeking a sense of self-worth and self-satisfaction, of acceptance and recognition. These people would rather be validated and recognized then tossed a bone. This is not to say, as a manager, a parent, or a partner, you should not learn to effectively combine internal and external rewards. Internal is longer lasting than external, but both are better than one.

A second consideration to understanding your audience is to disregard everything you've read or heard about personality types. Yes, there are some very valid books and theories that present various personality factors. Unfortunately though, real life does not produce exact measurable personality types that fit perfectly into pre-categorized boxes. Sure, we love to take personality tests. We love to see who the test results say we are. While these kinds of tests and quizzes are fun, and even sometimes enlightening and thought provoking, they cannot define us. We all have different backgrounds, experiences, perceptions, ideas, relationships, and educations. It would be impossible to take the highly complex personality of any one person and put him into a specific category, expecting to gain the ability to read him like a book.

You can, however, generalize. You can say that someone is, shy, loud, full of beans, hard to work with, friendly, or outlandish. You can, with relative safety, say something to that effect, realizing that the person you are saying it about might not always, under every circumstance, act the same way. For instance, you could take the most fun-loving, hysterical, clown of the classroom type of guy, steal his wallet and chances are, he won't be cracking too many jokes. People are people, not objects or pre-calculated machines. They run on their own constructs, complete with their own unique motivational drives and complex personality features.

For example, the clerk behind the counter at the electric company might seem reserved because she hates her job, but under that stern office demeanor, might reside a real party animal...who knows? The rule about classifying people is, *don't.* By paying attention to the approach that works best with the individuals you interact with most often will certainly take you farther in effective communications. When you incorporate the Effective Response Theory, however, you will improve all of your interactions, regardless of who the person is or how well you know them.

A book about effective communications of his nature would be remiss to not include at least a page or two on attitude. Your attitude is everything. It relates to who you are and how far you will go in this life. Your attitude shows through in virtually everything you do, and try as you may, your attitude, the way you feel about life in general, is pretty hard to hide. This being the case, it is important that you work often to improve your attitude and how you feel about yourself and others. Don't think for a moment that every interaction you have doesn't, in some way, shape, or form your present attitude for all the world to see. The rule is simple. The better your attitude is, the better your communication skills will be. If you feel good, it shows in your words, your actions, and your energy. People like to interact with people who have good attitudes; it's really that simple.

While we could go on for days about the important reasons behind acquiring a good attitude (or improving the one you already have), we are limited in time and space and the subject at hand is, after all, communications. Therefore, let's review what some of the well known "attitude experts" tell us about the importance of keeping our outlook bright. These experts have also clarified some of the very simple premises that help us get along better with others, as we will cover later on.

■■■

Famous for his many motivational contributions over several decades, Napoleon Hill is still well read and revered, worldwide. His thoughts about attitude were very specific and optimistically slanted, "A positive mind is key." Simply put, a positive mind is likely the most important ingredient to maintaining a healthy attitude.

Napoleon Hill offered an analogy long ago that is worthy of recall. He advises that we consider our minds like gardens; the flowers are good thoughts, and the weeds are negative thoughts. He told us if we made sure we always cared for our mental gardens, keeping our thoughts clean and optimistic and plucking up the weeds as they surfaced, we would go far to improve the quality of our attitudes, thus, our lives.

(Even today, Hill's books continue to sell and be recommended by scores of motivational speakers and writers. If you have never read, *Think and Grow Rich*, you are doing yourself a great disservice as it is inarguably the best personal development book ever written. In fact, I don't know of any self-help author or motivational speaker who hasn't read and promoted it.)

Understanding the "weed theory" proves that people recognize the powerful importance of how we manage our minds and our thoughts. More recent and more scientific in practice and delivery is Dr. Martin Seligman, Ph.D., who has spent his entire adult life researching and teaching psychology theories related to learned helplessness and optimism versus pessimism. In his book, *Learned Optimism*, he talks of his scientifically astute discoveries about pessimism, and outlines the disorder as follows:

- "Pessimism promotes depression
- Pessimism produces inertia rather than activity in the face of setbacks
- Pessimism is self-fulfilling
- Pessimism feels bad subjectively
- Pessimism is associated with poor physical health
- Pessimists are defeated when they try for high office
- Even when pessimists are right and things turn out badly, they still feel worse."

Dr. Seligman is a well-renowned and respected scientist. Yet for some reason when it comes to attitudes and emotions, the medical community has been slow to warm to the validity of such ideas. If you happen to be someone who doesn't recognize the important relationship your mental attitude has with your physical health, you might have to stretch your belief system a bit, but it is a stretch worth taking; one always affects the other.

Even though Dr. Seligman's list might seem somewhat harsh, think about the implications. If you know someone who is living a life of depression, or seems to possess any of these characteristics, how difficult is it to communicate with him or her? And even worse, what if it were you who was depressed or pessimistic?

The line between American bouts of depression and clinical depression are not always so easy to draw. Put another way, many of us face situations that drag us down. Moreover, most of us have days that deplete us or leave us short on energy and enthusiasm. Unfortunately, this is normal, and all but another sad societal reflection of life as we know it. However, when these feelings remain, become unmanageable, or tend to wreck your whole world, maybe it's time to seek outside support.

Even an emotionally healthy person can benefit from various forms of therapy, and certainly a person who suffers severe depression or other mental disorders should seek professional assistance. This is not to say that the whole world needs therapy (although it probably wouldn't hurt) but rather, there are times and situations when it is well warranted. Clearly, you can only control yourself, but at least that's a start. Beyond that, try to be cognizant when you spot depression in others— you will want to keep it in mind when you are knee deep in conversation with them. Remember though, this works the other way around too; people notice when you're not well tuned and chipper yourself.

Let's look at how this impacts our interactions.

The negativity associated with pessimism is clear. Think about how it hits you where you live. Wouldn't you rather converse and convene with happy spirits opposed to those that are down in the dumps? Unfortunately, we aren't always given an option. The best thing you can do for yourself and those you know, is keep your mind and attitude clean and positive. If you recognize yourself as someone who tends to see the pessimistic side of life, take steps to change it now; the impact will be dramatic.

It's not always easy to know if you exhibit negative thinking traits, but the quick quiz below will give you a hint. Remember, as noted earlier, there are no tests or exercises that can act as a panacea or tell-all. The exercises in this book are intended to serve as thought-provoking tools designed to assist you in laying fertile ground for positive interaction and self-improvement.

Optimistic Profile

1. Do you mentally criticize yourself?
2. When things go wrong, do you assume it's your fault?
3. When things go right, do you take credit for it?
4. Do you defend your negativity by explaining that you're more realistic than others?
5. Do you worry all the time?
6. Do you imagine the worst, or the best in any situation?
7. Do you suffer insomnia, or difficulty sleeping?
8. Do you often feel listless, hopeless, or sad for no explainable reason?

9. Do you always feel the need to be right in conversations?
10. Do you laugh more than you complain, or visa versa?

If you answered most or many of these questions in a manner that indicates you are pessimistic in your thinking, the good news is that you can reverse your thought patterns. People who think negative thoughts can improve the quality of their life by simply inserting more positive thoughts into their mind. For the questions above, generally speaking, people who are pessimistic tend to put themselves down, blame themselves when things go bad, but not take credit when they're good, worry too much, find the negative aspect in most situations, expect the worst, defend themselves aggressively, feel lethargic, and have trouble sleeping or want to sleep too much. Often times, these individuals will tell you they're not negative, just realistic.

Please understand that there is a difference between a mood and a constant state of mind. There are many times when someone in a bad mood might possess every negative trait listed, however, this does not necessarily make her a pessimistic person. We are all subject to grumpy moods; the challenge is to control it.

A study that was conducted demonstrated that one good way to improve your mood immediately was to "pretend" to be happy. Neuropyschologist Richard Hamilton, Ph.D. tells us, "The brain can't tell the difference between genuine, internal emotions and those that are imagined." He went on to say, "It secretes the appropriate chemicals in either case, so when you 'imagine' upbeat thoughts, the brain responds by boosting its production of serotonin and other chemicals linked to happiness."

So how do you use this information to help you? For starters, assume a positive stance and state of mind when are you interacting with others, according to this and additional studies, not only will you feel and seem more optimistic in your interactions, but the positive mind-set may very well "rub" off on the person you are communicating with. When we maintain a positive attitude and optimistic thinking, it cannot help but affect our interaction in a productive manner. Beyond that, and still keeping the study in mind, if you assume a positive demeanor, you'll actually start to *feel* it for real!

While you can address your own attitude and work to keep it positive, it is not always easy to contend with someone else who is negative. Clearly, the best thing you can do is to start by understanding and accepting their perspective. You cannot take responsibility for changing it and you cannot, no matter what you do, control the way another person feels. Moreover, you cannot control the way another person reacts, what she says, or how she says it. This means it is up to you to ensure you have taken care of your own role in the interaction. Your own role consists of maintaining a positive attitude and practicing the Effective Response Theory that follows.

In summary on attitude, there is clear indication that the way we feel about our lives and ourselves affects our health, our outlook on life, and undoubtedly, our interactions with others. Our interactions will benefit when we feel good about who we are and what we're doing. It is inevitable that the power of our own positive nature will have a pleasing impact on others and take us closer to our goals. So smile and sparkle from the inside out, or visa versa, if that be the case, and begin to enjoy the life you have.

ETHICS

Finally, we need to have a quick review on the importance of ethics in communications. You cannot communicate effectively if you don't tell the truth. While business might call for some periodic sidestepping or confidential communications, there is never any acceptable reason for lying. Not being truthful is deceptive and destructive to personal and professional interactions. If you are forbidden to say something or sworn to secrecy, there are ways to express that fact without lying and without divulging any confidential information.

Consider the degree of importance the law puts on telling the truth. Committing perjury is a federal offense. Regardless of how advanced we become with technology, space travel or medicine, we still put our hand on the bible and swear to tell the truth in a court of law. Being honest is not an option. When you fail to speak the truth, you are not only betraying those around you, you are betraying yourself. There is no honor in lying. We are all guilty of telling the occasional "white lie;" a fib that appears to hurt no one, at least at face value. Evidence of this can be found in the elementary-aged child who tells the teacher the dog ate his homework. But is it really harmless?

Only you can be the judge of your own acts of honesty, but ask yourself some questions before you utter any lies. For instance, who is the lie, or fib protecting? Often times we might not tell the truth to avoid hurting someone's feelings. This is generally a selfless kind of act, and one that women are infamous for. If your friend is wearing a dress that you find ridiculously tight, and she asks you what you think of it, there is no need to hurt her feelings. However, you don't need to go overboard in the other direction either.

If something is glaringly wrong and someone asks for your honest opinion, you owe it to yourself and the other person to tell the truth. That doesn't mean that you cannot couch the truth, should it be negative, between kindness and compassion. For example, with your friend who had the overly tight dress, you might tell her yes, you like it. But then she presses you, says she is thinking about wearing it to a big office event where she wants to make a good impression, should she wear it?

Telling your friend the dress is fine when she casually asks your opinion and you want to avoid needlessly hurting her feelings is fine. When more is at stake, however, and she's asking for your honest input, you would be remiss to lie. Naturally, you don't have to tell her that her gut is sticking out and it looks horrendous. You could say that you don't think it's professional enough to make the kind of impression she is looking for. You could suggest another dress you've seen her wear before. The point is, that nearly all of us are put on the spot from time to time in a way that makes us feel uncomfortable. We don't want to tell lies, yet we don't want to hurt other people's feelings. Here is where ethics, coupled with a compassionate heart, will pay off. Avoid hurting someone's feelings if there is any way around it, and there usually is. However, being candid is a quality that all honorable people possess, and there is never any honor in being a liar.

Polly Young Eisenprath writes, in her book, *Women and Desire*, "When we tell the truth to a partner or a friend, we are indeed vulnerable to being judged, blamed, or rejected." And this is true. What scares us about telling our friend her dress is too tight, or our partner his belly is too big is less about hurting their feelings than it is about risking rejection on our part. Sure, we don't want to see someone we care about feel bad or sad or dissatisfied with her self, however, an even stronger force is the one that tells us we must make certain everybody loves us. Sometimes, we have to take chances. Be honest in your interactions, albeit coated with love and compassion. Telling the truth is only one part of the picture.

Ethical communications would also preclude threatening, bribing, and over-promising. In any business or personal relationship, it is easy to black mail. It's not that we're inherently deceptive human beings, it's just that bribery and incentives are very closely related. This is especially true when we are inundated with the importance of motivation and positive reinforcement. We are taught that rewarding our children, our employees, and our clients for good actions is a good thing. So when does it turn into bribery?

If you are talking to an associate on the phone, telling him about a new plan you would like to have him buy into, and that one of the benefits would be some exclusive opportunity that he would otherwise miss out on, that is an incentive. However, if you're talking to the same associate about the same project, but injecting a perk that is in no way related to the subject at hand...that might be construed as bribery.

Consider the following examples and you will better see the point.

Manager: *Hey Bob, this is a great program. As a matter of fact, anyone who signs up now is guaranteed free shipping once a month.*

Or:

Manager: *Hey Bob, this is a great program. As a matter of fact, if you'd like to sign up now, I just might be willing to call Joe about the other deal we spoke of last week.*

The two examples are fairly clear in differentiating the merits between an incentive and a bribe. Generally speaking, you should limit your inspirations with incentives, as opposed to bribes. This doesn't mean that most of Corporate America, or the political arena (or any other arena for that matter), necessarily abides by this rule, but that is beside the point. Remember, you can only control your own words and actions, not those of others. Doing or saying something you know is wrong, because you see other people do it, is no excuse. What comes around goes around, and if you don't approach all of your interactions with others from a very ethical platform, it is sure to catch up with you someday.

Now that we've looked at some of the primary ways we cast a negative light on our interactions with others, it's time to explore the act of effective communications. Before starting though, make a point to recall the areas you've noted in yourself that can stand a bit of improvement and then work on a daily basis to rid yourself of communication flaws or negative reactions that might benefit from your efforts.

Exercise:

The area(s) I need to work on most when it comes to my interactions with others is:

_____

_____

_____

_____

I notice I do this most with (list the people or kinds of people):

_____

_____

_____

_____

I will remind myself by:

_____

_____

_____

_____

YOUR GOALS ARE GOLD

Now the bright side of getting along better with the rest of the world. As with anything, eliminating an unwanted element is always easier when you have something good to replace it with. The Effective Response Theory is just such a thing.

This theory is not some fancy, scholarly, pie-in-the-sky idea that would take a graduate degree in order to understand. Quite the contrary, it could, in its simplest terms, be reduced to common sense. Even common sense, however, is easier to apply when it's been mapped out and presented in a logical manner. The Effective Response Theory (ERT) starts with understanding the negative reaction portion that we've been discussing so far, and gives us something more productive to replace it with. We started out by understanding that the words we say to others, and they to us, are often not effective because they are *reactionary* instead of *responsive*. When this happens, we are often communicating from our egos and insecurities instead of from our hearts and heads. Let's consider the productive portion of this interaction-equation.

ERT is a step-by-step formula that will increase the success of your interactions with others. Primarily, it consists of responding instead of reacting, and there are sure steps to ensure that you do just that. In a nutshell, the Theory consists of identifying goals, stepping outside of the scene, walking in the other person's shoes, asking questions and listening to answers, empathizing, and finally, responding. When you start to apply these techniques in your daily life, you'll wonder how you ever interacted without them.

Not only will you be considered a much easier person to talk to, you will be highly revered and find it incredibly easy to accomplish your goals with the support and assistance that the rest of the world is happy to give you.

You will learn the power of positive communications.

GOAL IDENTITY

*T*HE very first step in ERT is to identify your interaction goals. If you are a manager and want to have a paper revised and edited by your assistant, then that becomes the goal. What tends to happen with most of us is that we get caught up in the ego/insecurity portion of our interactions and forget what we set out to do in the first place.

If you start out with your goal in mind you are instantly aware of what direction you want the interaction to take and be well aware when it takes a wrong turn. It is only through this awareness that you will be able to keep the conversation on a productive path.

We have noted repeatedly that there are two ways to communicate: productively and non-productively. If you intend to achieve productivity in your interactions you're going to have to start out by identifying exactly what productivity means to you. Sales people are well skilled in this area. They may meander in the conversation, but their eye is always on the carrot. They are constantly aware that they are on the road to closing the deal and they pay special attention to the sign posts along the way, rarely venturing too far off the productive path.

By identifying your goal before conversations or interactions begin, you are better equipped to keep your communications on the right road. Not coincidentally, our goals start forming well before our mouths ever open. The earlier these goals are identified, the stronger the likelihood that we will reach them. There are three kinds of goals we will look at. They are independent, yet interwoven. Or, perhaps a better term would be "progressive," as one kind of goal usually expands into the next.

Our personal and professional goals account for the first group of goal-setting efforts. While jotting down your goals may not seem at all related to your communication efforts, take heart. Defining who we are and where we are going in life has everything to do with how we get there. If you want to become president of your company, your interactions and communications with those you work with will be instrumental to your success. Furthermore, if you are making an effort to be a better parent, your communications with off springs will certainly be a key factor of consideration.

The purpose is not to track goals and monitor accomplishments simply for the sake of success itself. It is instead to ensure that our interactions are in direct alignment with our life goals. If you wish to become a politician, your interactions with key people will make or break your plans. In this context our goals are very much related to our communication efforts. This is the only level of goal setting that you need to document. The other levels will be assessed and applied on an instantaneous, as-occurring basis.

Take time now to truly understand what it is you are ultimately after. Whether it is personal (getting along better with partner), or professional (getting a promotion), by writing it down, you make it real. All too often we sail through life constantly hitting our head against brick walls, not getting anywhere worthwhile, or getting there, bruised upon arrival. It might seem like you are constantly barraged with those who appear to be standing in the way of your success. Unfortunately, it is our failure to interact effectively that truly stands in our way, and that's something we are all capable of changing.

When we recognize what it is we are after, it becomes much easier to stay on communication-track. In other words, it will always serve you well to remember *why* you are doing what it is you are doing, and then act accordingly. When you identify your communication goals, both long-term and short-term, you are more likely to stay on a path that will help you see them through to completion. If you don't think setting goals seems like it has much to do with the efficacy of your communication skills, consider the following example:

Let's say your goal is to teach English Literature at a very prestigious university. You know you have less of an education than the other applicants. On the way to the interview, a careless college kid trips you and causes your papers to fly all over the place. The Professor who will interview you is standing nearby. Now while this is a seemingly innocuous scenario, think about it.

Even if you were not on your way to an important interview, a careless kid colliding into you would send even the most optimistic person to the far right. You might not necessarily yell, but you would certainly let that student know that you didn't appreciate his act of flying into you at warp speed. Fair enough? So generally speaking, the best of us might tend to react a little negatively to such a situation.

However, because you have already pre-determined your goal, to get the job, you are thinking of how your interactions, not only with the professor, but also with one of the professor's students (the one who ran you over), might impact that ultimate goal.

By handling the run-in with the student in an authoritative, but pleasantly accepting manner you have shown the professor that you are quite capable of effectively communicating with students who tend to do clumsy things. The way you handled this interaction had the potential of taking you closer toward or farther from the goal you set for yourself.

The logical explanation as to why our written goals possess power probably lies in the fact that once we've written something down, we've made it official; taken it seriously. In our mind's eye, it becomes a reality the minute we jot it down, and then it's our natural sub-conscious tenancy to manifest it for real. The merits of goal setting are enormous and span well beyond communication skills. In addition to helping you keep on track with more effective interactions, consider the great value you can add to your life by setting goals for yourself in your personal and professional life.

When you write something down, you set it in motion. If you've not yet identified your primary goals in life, perhaps now is as good a time as any to get busy. Use the following page to document your goals. This way, you will always have your plans on paper, and your map close at hand. It is easier to respond effectively, even with troubled or conflicting communications, when we remember who we are and where we're going.

GOALS 101

My ultimate goal for my professional life is:

_____

_____

_____

_____

I will accomplish this by:

_____

_____

_____

_____

My ultimate goal for my personal life is:

_____

_____

_____

_____

I will accomplish this by:

_____

_____

_____

_____

Now it's time to look at the ways we apply goal setting specifically to our interactions with others. These are not goals you must write down in advance or at all for that matter. These are the goals that exist in every single interaction that ever occurs. Your role when you communicate, whether it is to simply obtain directions or win a debate, is driven by two kinds of goals. Often times we fail to recognize these goals, which take us farther from them.

An "end goal" is the overall, long term goal we have for that particular interaction or communications. For example, maintaining someone as a client, would be an end goal, hence, whenever we interact with that person we will be sure to keep our communication efforts in alignment with the goal of keeping him as a client. When you communicate with someone on a limited basis, say the dry cleaning clerk or a bank teller, usually an end goal is all that exists for that specific interaction. The end goal might be to retrieve the dry cleaning, withdraw cash from your savings account, or something similar that has a purpose easy to identify. While these one-time interactions are simple to spot, don't be fooled into thinking that there's no room for improvement.

For instance, when you park your car at the dry cleaner, your goal is fairly obvious; you want to pick up your clothes. Even a mundane errand such as this could put your communication skills to the test.

For instance, add to this scenario the fact that you've only got a few minutes before you need to pick your son up from soccer practice. You enter the dry cleaners and the line of people waiting to be served circles two city blocks. Or, say there is no line, but the couldn't-care-less clerk mentions that your best suit was ruined, 'so sorry.'

These are just a couple of examples of how an ordinary, no-problem-piece-of- cake communication could rake you over the coals. But you've got your end goal planted in your mind, right? Since you already know your end goal is to pick up your clothes, you're going to keep your ego on the other side of town. For instance, when you see the line is too long to wait…pushing your way to the front and cursing at the clerk isn't going to make you reach your goal any sooner. Further, if your suit isn't ready, reaching over the counter and strangling the messenger probably isn't going to manifest your Sunday- Best any quicker.

When we keep our end goals in mind it assists us in our effort to remain calm and in control, which isn't so easy in a world that is often anything but. We noted specific situations above that tend to cause reactions (instead of responses) in many of us. Now let's review the actual oral efforts in a similar circumstance. You're in a hurry, you stop at the dry cleaner and they tell you they can't find the suit that you plan on wearing to a presentation the next day.

Recall the saying that Abe Lincoln is credited with, "You can catch more flies with honey…" Yes, the saying is old, but fortunately, the flies don't mind. People simply respond more favorably to you if you're nice. So when you're at the dry cleaner and the young clerk flippantly informs you that she can't find your four-hundred-dollar suit, don't yell.

Instead, recall your end goal is to get the suit. It often becomes easy to replace our end goal with new goals, such as, to show that person how much smarter, wiser, more powerful, or plain foolish we can be. This is what happens when you see someone yelling at a clerk behind the counter at a shoe store because she won't take back the worn tennis shoes without a receipt. It really isn't about the receipt— it's about the manner in which the lack of receipt is presented. Really. So, instead of losing site of your goal to get your dry cleaning from point A to point B, your car, remember to keep your goal in mind. Ask smart questions in a wise way.

Could the suit be misfiled in the many rows of dry cleaning? Can we check to see if there's anything on file? Could it have lost the tag and be in the non-claimed section? For every situation you come across there will be smart questions you can ask. When you ask smart questions and make perceptive suggestions, the person you are interacting with will be much more responsive and willing to assist. Besides that, when you remember to respond, rather than react, people will like you more and won't call you nasty names when you turn to walk away. The most important aspect, however, is to remember that when you respond instead of react, you are closer to reaching your goal. Think of it this way: if your goals are a destination and your communications a vehicle, when you react negatively, it's like hitching a ride from the other side of town, whereas, when you respond effectively, it's like getting dropped off right at the corner. It takes you so much closer.

Essentially, your end goals are the *purpose of the communication*. When we forget the purpose of the interaction, we fail to maintain focus. When this happens, we allow the potential of our negative reactions to take over the conversation.

The key to this chapter and this first vital step of ERT, is to ask yourself in literally all of your communication efforts, the following question:

Is this taking me closer to my goal?

It is only when we fail to consider the ultimate goal of the interaction at hand that we allow our egos and insecurities to speak up in our stead. Even if your goal is simply to keep the peace with an annoying relative, that is in itself a goal—it is an end goal. To clarify, there is one more goal that plays a role in your interactions.

The third kind of goal that usually occurs with our more frequent communications is called a "mini goal " Mini goals are the ones we tend to overlook the most, yet they tend to have the greatest impact in our day-to-day interactions with the people that are most important in our lives.

A mini goal is an immediate goal and often refers to a conflict or "bump in the road" of your end goal. See if you can identify the mini goal in the example below:

You're ready to close a deal with a very important client. You've worked hard and long to make this transaction a reality. There is one more sales point you need to make before you're sure he'll sign the dotted line, but he just informed you that he's got to get to the airport or he'll miss his flight.

Did you spot it? Going one step backward, let's point out the obvious. Closing the deal is your end goal. Getting the client to sign the contract will make your end goal a reality. Now though, there appears to be a cog in the wheel. That's a good way to describe mini goals; they are cogs in the wheel that must be addressed before attaining the end goal.

In our example above the fact that the client has to catch a plane before you've completed your pitch is a problem. Your mini goal would be to fix it. Do you see the difference in the two levels of goals?

The first level, the end-goal, is to close the sale. The second level, or mini goal, is to rectify the airport situation so that you can make your end goal happen.

Dividing up and identifying end goals and mini goals can help you maintain focus on what really matters. It is when we lose site of these goals that our interactions tend to crumble. Consider this common occurrence in the real estate industry. An agent lists a property. The end goal would be to sell the house, yes? Undoubtedly, this is a challenging goal in and of itself, however, often times, a dozen or more conflicts will arise that present the agent to consider mini goals as a means to an end.

For example, it is not at all unusual in this scenario for the seller of the property to call the agent and suggest that the property might have been listed at too low of a selling price. This is common in real estate because sellers tend to think their property is worth more than the market will bear. When this client calls, complaining about the pricing, the agent then has a mini goal: to reassure the client that the property is priced correctly for the current market. If the agent were to forget his end goal, to sell the listing, then this bump in the road could easily cause the interaction to result in a negative reaction, in which case, he might lose the listing.

By identifying the end goal of selling the property, and then the mini goal of reassuring his client the house is priced right, the agent can ensure that every word he utters in the conversation is in direct alignment with both of his goals. Remember, communications are either productive or non-productive. For clarification, those communications that are productive are the ones that drive us closer to our goals. Conversely, it is when we overlook our goals that interactions take a non-productive turn.

To wrap this chapter up, let's consider an example that starts with professional goals and expands into the mini goal of an interaction. While your mind will race to figure out the correct response to the dilemma, don't. The purpose of this example is not for you to determine what you would do in the same instance. It is instead designed to enable you to recognize the different levels of goals as they might apply in real life. When you have read through the scenario, answer the questions beneath it.

Sara works in an advertising firm. Her professional goal is to become the Creative Director. She has worked diligently, acquired the education, taken every project that's been passed her way and worked late hours, all toward making her goal a reality. Phil is the owner of the firm and the person ultimately responsible for Sara's promotion. Rita, a competitor for the same position, doesn't always play by the rules. Rita has been known to cause trouble for anyone who stands in her way, and has made it very clear she plans on getting the position.

Phil has asked Sara to prepare a special storyboard for a big client. Sara is ecstatic about the opportunity. She spends all weekend working on the project and is only missing one key component that she determines she can insert first thing Monday morning.

When she arrives at the office bright and early Monday morning, storyboard in hand, she inquires about the missing piece of her presentation. Rita, she learns, is the only person who has access to the file.

Now see if you can identify these goals:

1) What is Sara's long-term professional goal?

What is Sara's end goal?

What is Sara's mini goal?

If you said that Sara's professional goal was to be a Creative Director, and you should have—since it's stated in the first paragraph—bingo. Number two would be the project at hand. Sara's end goal is to complete the storyboard so that Phil will is impressed and she increases her chance at winning the promotion. The third answer, the mini goal, is to obtain the information that only Rita can access. Do you see that if the first two goals are not kept in mind, things might really get thrown out of whack? If Sara is to secure the file from Rita, she's going to need to keep her goals foremost in her mind, lest Rita's competitiveness and lack of cooperation might knock her right off course.

This is only one of at least two million scenarios that might offer you insight into the three levels of goal setting. The point to glean from all of this is that often times our interactions include more than one layer of goals and that by identifying them, we are better able to stay focused and in alignment with them.

Your long term goal, both personal and professional, should be held in your mind, each and every day. This becomes easy when you write your goals down and post them in a place that you can see them often.

So while your long term goal is always on your mind, all you will need to do is recall the accompanying goals that help you on your way, then speak and act to that end. The best way to act in accordance to the goals you have set for yourself is to automatically bring them to mind with each particular interaction. Every time you enter a conversation, consider what the end goal is. Perhaps it is nothing more than to say hello to a co-worker or share closeness with a child. However, when you immediately identify the goal, you will be that much more prepared if and when a mini goal rears it's needy head.

Productive interactions begin with defining goals.

Chapter Nine
STEPPING OUT

THE next component of ERT pertains to our ability to step outside of any situation for an instant assessment. A quick caveat: during heated discussions or conflicting communications, it's not always easy to remove oneself from the moment. This though, is the very reason it's vital. We're going to learn to eliminate the emotions long enough to assess the situation.

Some interactions and communications allow us the luxury of time. For example, you might hear a message in your voice mail, receive a letter or an email, or be asked to "get back" to someone with a response. In these kinds of situations you are much more able to step outside of the situation and make a logical assessment prior to, and instead of, blurting out an inappropriate reaction. Coincidentally, when it is the other extreme (you have to respond immediately, and perhaps impromptu), when the interactions might be emotionally packed, this stepping outside of the situation brings the most benefit. Unfortunately though, it is the kinds of interactions we could use the extra cool down time, when seem to be allotted the least. When we have time to think and assess, we generally go through a ritual that allows us to get all of the "garbage" out of the way and ultimately come back with the kind of response that is most effective in taking us closer towards our goals.

The good news is that with a little effort, practice and understanding, you can learn to step outside of the situation and become a much more effective communicator, even without the luxury of extra time to mull things over. When you are in the middle of a heated debate you generally don't find yourself with the option nor inclination to say, "Let me just get back to you on that." Although, it would do many of us well, to be sure.

For the sake of clarity, let's define exactly what we mean when we refer to "stepping outside of the situation."

To step outside of a situation is to view it as an outsider looking only at the facts. You would be amazed if you considered how much emotional baggage is usually attached to your most heated discussion. Certain words or actions can trigger off buried emotions before you even know what hits you. By learning to step outside of the situation, you can focus more analytically on the communication at hand.

Stepping outside of the situation involves a few key elements that you'll want to become familiar with and apply to your own interaction efforts. Humility is important. Being humble voids much of the ego at work and makes us stronger communicators. Next, we must remember that our ability to control others is non-existent. It is only when we understand and accept this fact fully that we can apply our attention toward improvement where it really belongs, on ourselves. Finally, the biggest and most productive act that any of us can learn in any kind of interaction we take part in is the art of not taking things too personally. There is surely a fine line between constructive feed back versus unwarranted criticism, and learning to differentiate between the two is paramount. Here we learn that anything someone else thinks or says to or about us is only their opinion and we cannot let it color our communication efforts.

In his book, *The Four Agreements*, Ruiz spells out some of the most powerful interaction actions we could ever hope to learn. Learning to not take things personally is one that can help you in all of your interactions and relationships. It is so easy to find fault in another, but heaven forbid if someone finds fault in us. It is our human nature to need acceptance, regardless of what we do. This is a poignant fact. We all need to feel accepted. Unfortunately, people are people and it is our nature as such to not always agree or approve of what others do. The key is to not dwell on those opinions as law.

Certainly there will be times in your life and your career where good constructive feedback can serve you well. You might be delicately pointed toward a part of yourself or your efforts that require improvement for increased productivity. You might have a certain fault that, once removed, will dramatically enhance your performance or relationship potential. There are, however, many more times that are much more frequent when people will say things to you that have no business even entering your mind.

Learning to not take things personally is vital to the success of your effective communication skills. All too often our own insecurity, matched with someone else's over-active ego or insecurity, can set the stage for self-defeat. Someone says something out of anger or insecurity and you interpret it to be true. When this is negative, as it often is, you will tend to react rather than respond. When you react, it is not going to be productive to your goals or to relationship at hand.

Learning to not take things personally is a big part of this particular step in ERT. Without acquiring this ability, you will not be able to step outside of the situation; you will be too busy worrying about something someone said to you and wondering if it's true. After reading the first section of this book, you should be better attuned to the way we all tend to react in relation to our ego. Once you understand the premise that most of us are continuously dealing with our own set of insecurities, and often interact from that foundation, it becomes easier to overlook negative reactions in others. We can begin to understand that it is them reacting to their own issues, which we sometimes get stuck in the middle of. It helps substantially if we recognize the person that has said or done something to us, even if it was done or said in complete contempt, does not have the power to change how we feel about ourselves. Taken one step farther, the person who uses cruel or unjust words cannot *cause* you to use the same kind of words in response. A common example of this follows.

One person is in a terrible mood, maybe very busy, under stress, or just plain grumpy. The other person does something that doesn't set quite right with him and all heck breaks lose. For example, say Bill is getting a lot of pressure to finish a report that technically no human being could finish in the period of time that has been allotted. You walk by singing the latest soundtrack from a new Nicolas Cage movie and he all but bites your head off, "Do you always have to sing that irritating crap?" He asks, glaring through his glasses.

In this instance, you have a couple of choices as to how you will respond, but right now we're not at all concerned with your response. Here we are learning how to let the negative stuff roll right off your back. A lot of people in this situation would give serious consideration to putting a muzzle on their musical expression from that day forward.

Most human beings, given the same set of circumstances, would feel offended; they would take it personally. The trick is to realize that people snap, attack and strike out, and sometimes you just happen to be right in the line of fire. Think of it as passing a rattlesnake on the road; stay out of the way and walk on by. Don't fight back; just get out.

Another way to say this is that regardless of how poorly a person interacts with you or speaks toward you, they cannot force you to react negatively unless you choose to do so. Often, it is the times when we feel insulted, threatened or injured that we do best to practice the art of not taking things personally. People are people and sometimes they say and do things that they should not say or do. You cannot base your interactions on another person's mistakes. If you react negatively because someone said something that was not appropriate or kind you have put yourself on the same level as that person. How can this be effective?

Taking things personally is very common and something we all fall prey to. Now that you understand all about ego and insecurity, you should be able to identify that most people who react negatively are really acting out of fear. It isn't personal. Yet somehow, humans that we are, being put down in the middle of an intense emotional outburst makes us feel like we're being attacked.

Consider one more example: You are a salesperson for a big paper supply company. You visit a client, one that is known to fly off the handle now and then. When you walk in the door he practically accosts you, saying that her card stock order is two days late. You make the appropriate follow up phone call right then and there. You learn that the paper has been shipped but it's two days late because it was on backorder, something no one told you about. You have done your job, you have remained cool, and maybe even bitten your tongue while this customer was reacting negatively and putting you down. Say he tells you he thinks you handled things inappropriately and that you that you are by far the worst salesperson he has ever seen.

This would obviously be difficult for even the best of us to not take personally. Even though we know, at least on an intellectual level, that this person is reacting irrationally and that we are not wrong in our actions. We know the customer is angry and has a reputation for being difficult anyway. You know you are not the first salesperson he has orally insulted. Hopefully, it goes without saying, that you never need to force yourself to stay in a situation where you are being attacked. In this example however, the customer is more of a hot head, grumbling at life in general, and you just happen to be his target.

You leave the store. You forget, soon enough, that he was mad about his late order; he's just being a difficult customer and everyone has had the same kind of experience with him. The one thing you can't shake though is his comment about your being the lousiest salesperson he's ever seen. Why is that? Essentially, it is because we all are fairly apt at intellectualizing ourselves out of some things, but other things, those that have an emotional impact, become more challenging.

You know you are not a lousy salesperson. Perhaps you have an award on the wall that says so. The point is, when someone attacks you in a vulnerable spot, you will internalize it, no matter what. This doesn't require a heated debate to feel like one just took place. Even in casual conversation someone can say something to you that you find painful. You will internalize and dwell upon a comment that was forgotten by the person who said it just as soon as it was said.

Learning to not take things personally is important to your interactions with others and especially important to your interactions with self. To address this issue from a logical perspective will help you understand how and why you must adapt the ability to not internalize what others say to or about you.

In the example of being called a lousy salesperson, consider the choices. You could go home, have a bad weekend, dwell on it and let it otherwise impact your performance. Will that change anything? Will beating yourself up or obsessing over a statement that was made, that you know wasn't true to begin with, have any positive results? Of course not. It will not change the fact that the statement was made in the first place (remember, you can't "unyell"), nor will it serve you any practical purpose to dwell on a negative untruth about yourself.

The unfortunate part about internalizing negative comments from others is that we tend to wallow in the aftermath when the person who said it has all but forgotten the conversation ever took place. Yes, sometimes people acknowledge that they say mean things and perhaps

93

they even apologize later, however, *you* have to take enough responsibility to not let things that other people say impact your life in a negative manner. No one should have that power. Understand that nothing will change the fact that the customer called you a lousy salesperson. But understand also, that you have the option of not accepting the words as true, especially when they were intended to harm.

Learning to not take things personally is an on-going effort in our interaction experiences. There will always be things that people say, either innocently or intentionally, that tend to bring us down. When we learn to let it slide, not let it consume us, we will be much better equipped to step outside the situation and remain humble.

Being humble isn't always easy. An action that is almost directly opposite of our need to be right is being humble. Not feeling compelled to let everyone know how good we are or how much more we know about something is tough. This is particularly true when we feel that we are being challenged, whether it's real or imagined. Being humble means that you don't have to "prove" yourself in your communications. When you are not being humble, chances are that your ego has taken over. Inevitably, this means that you are not interacting in alignment with your goals. Recall that productive communication involves responding effectively and is always in alignment with your goals, whereas non-productive communication involves negative reaction and usually drives you *away* from your goals.

As human beings, being humble is probably our biggest challenge. Yet, ironically, it is always those who possess and demonstrate the epitome of humility that we are most drawn to. Notice our respect for some of the most humble people who have walked the face of the Earth: Jesus, Mahatma Gandhi and Mother Theresa, for example. These are people able to step outside of the situation in order to do what they think is right. That's what being humble is all about.

If you can master the art of humility, at least to some degree, you will find your interactions improve tremendously. The reason for this is primarily psychological in nature, yet very easy to understand. Think of each person as being divided into two parts. There is the ego side and the humble side. We each possess these two sides that operate from different platforms. Not only do they operate from different platforms, they *speak* different languages. Let's call one language "ego talk," and the other, "humble heart."

When we react negatively to something someone has said, we are speaking ego talk. We are addressing the other individual from our own ego and insecurities. The other person automatically recognizes the language. "Oh, she speaks ego talk, okay, I know that dialect," and the problems ensue. We begin carrying on a conversation that is negative in construct and cannot possibly lead us to a productive outcome.

When you operate from a humble heart it's reflected in your words, your tone and your demeanor. Even for a person who is speaking ego talk, the presence of humble heart will cause the ego to eventually run out of fuel; there is no contest. Developing a more humble outlook and assuming humility in your dealings with others will take you many miles toward improved interactions.

People cannot help but be nice to you when you are humble. Often times, they check their ego at the door. Generally speaking, this is because those who are humble do not threaten others. People do not consider you as someone who hits below the belt or attempts to usurp their goals. People feel better when they deal with humble beings because they know there is no hidden agenda that they must look out for.

In direct relation with being humble comes the realization that we cannot control others. For some reason, part of being human, at least in this century and society, means that we need to feel in charge of something. Perhaps it is our own lack of self-esteem that propels this need, yet it is everywhere we look. Even small children exhibit it by "parenting" toys, pets, siblings, or other children. Next to being right, we like to be boss.

Our ego self that compels us to run the show often fails to see the one simple truth about human nature: We can't control anyone but ourselves. That doesn't mean we cannot order, insist, direct, command, or instruct another individual. It simply means that we never truly have complete dominion over another person.

In his landmark book, *Man's Search for Meaning,* Dr. Viktor Frankel tells us about his horrific experience in a Nazi war camp. The premise of his work was to explain how some people in the camp survived and others did not. With all conditions being equal, Dr. Frankel correctly surmised that the primary difference between those who survived and those who did not was the *will* to live. Maybe some had families that they believed were still alive and they needed to live long enough to reunite. Frankel's study shows us that when we are stripped of everything humanly possible, physically and/or emotionally, we are still in control of our will. It is not possible to change a person's mind unless the person allows it. We cannot control other people.

Dr. Frankel's work was revolutionary, yet most of us fail to reap the message deeply enough to apply it to our own lives for our own benefit and the benefit of others. We simply cannot control what another person thinks. Parents often fall prey to this error. Consider how many parents attempt to tell their children what they should think and how they should feel. This simply does not work and often times will create an effect opposite of the one desired.

Understanding that you cannot control what another person thinks should be a tremendous relief. For once you realize you're only responsible for yourself, you are freed up to concentrate on improving your own efforts, not everyone else's.

We understand that there are some things about other people that we control to the extent that we are responsible for their actions. A parent is responsible for child care and safety, making sure the homework gets done and disciplining as needed. A manager is responsible for ensuring goals are met, budgets are kept and employees are productive. There is, however, a difference between controlling and being responsible for a situation. When we attempt the impossible, controlling what the other person thinks, says or feels, we are looking for trouble.

The need to control others is the perfect partner to the need to be right. We don't need either. As a matter of fact, when we learn to let both of these go, our interactions improve immensely, so do our relationships and our stress levels. Often times we find ourselves in heated debates that, when reduced down to size, are really nothing more than our need to control the situation. Our ego butting into our interaction.

To improve this overpowering element, spend some time thinking about the last heated discussion you took part in. Identify the situation and think about why you needed to be in control. What was at stake if you lost that self-imposed need for control? It is only through thought-provoking self-exploration and real life analysis that we can overcome our need to control others. Consider this example and note whether or not you see yourself or someone you might know in the characters.

Jane and Mary are working on a project together. Jane is overseeing the budget and Mary the implementation. The project is to increase teddy bear sales in their toy division by the end of the year. Jane has come up with a feasible plan that breaks down expenditures over the four-month period they are working in. When Mary sees the budget, she automatically feels as if she has lost control. She interprets Jane's efforts as trying to "take over" the project and even stepping into Mary's territory. The conversation might go something like this.

Jane: *So if we maintain a monthly budget of $1,280, we can safely stay within range.*

Mary: *Well, one campaign I'm considering is going to run at least $1,600.*

Jane: *Okay, so we cut back on another month.*

Mary: *I think this would work best if I told you my plans and then you worked the budget around it.*

Can't you just feel Mary's insecurity in the pit of your stomach? How often do you or someone you know react the same way to something that was completely benign to begin with?

Again, this is just one simple, everyday example of how we feel compelled to keep in control of those things we find ourselves involved with. In this scenario, the objective should have been for the two individuals to work in sync so that they could produce profitable and productive results. Instead, in an effort to keep some kind of imaginary control Mary is spending precious time and energy, not to mention creating communication disaster, on something that is counter-productive to the task at hand.

We all do this. We like an idea just fine if it is ours. The minute someone else tries to take credit or offer instruction, we feel almost instantly compelled to go in the opposite direction. We like to be in control. Even children, craving independence, are commonly overheard saying "Let me try, I want to do it!"

This drive to control, however, can be used to our benefit when the person we try to control is our self. It is never productive and always futile to waste time trying to control the thoughts, words or actions of other people. Directly related, and perhaps more challenging, is learning to not take things personally.

When you learn how to not take the utterances of others personally, and you begin practicing the art of being humble, you are in a far better position to excel at your communication skills. You will not risk allowing your ego or insecurities to take over and mar your efforts. Learn to let the negative things that people say roll off of your back and interact from a humble heart. Only entertain the possibility of truth when the words were not said in anger and they somehow resonate in a useful and productive way. Even where constructive feedback is concerned, make sure the source is indeed qualified to give it. For instance, if Joe is dishing up his unsolicited opinion on how you should implement your next career move, and Joe has never held a job for more than two months, you'd probably be better off calling the psychic hotline than you would be following advice from Joe.

This isn't to imply that sometimes the answers we seek don't come from unexpected places. Hence the adage, *"Out of the mouths of babes."* This can primarily be attributed to the fact that us grown ups like to intellectualize ourselves to oblivion, often losing sight of the obvious issues at hand. Then along comes a four-year old who can see the answer clearly. With this in mind, there is no pat answer to whom you should trust for good solid advice. Most certainly though, you should trust yourself.

Learning to let go of what other people say or think about you is a huge step. It means you are walking on a tightrope all alone. Putting yourself on the line though and taking full responsibility for your words and your actions and not letting them be negatively colored by others is one of the most liberating things you will ever do. Once you learn to detach from detrimental talk and opinion you will be better armed to pursue your interactions to the winning end. Further, it will allow you to easily progress past this step of seeing beyond the situation by looking at it objectively.

Learning to step outside the situation requires you to remove all ego-aspects of the interaction. It allows you to assess the situation without the clutter of personal opinions and emotions that so often cloud our communicative efforts. In order to effectively perform this step, you will need to strip all real or imagined hidden agendas. You will need to consider the situation from a purely analytical point of view.

It is often amazing at how differently situations look when they are not jaded with our own emotional agenda. When we remove our ego and insecurities from the situation, it appears in a whole new light. It also becomes easier to understand the role we play in making or breaking the interaction.

Let's take the earlier example of Mary and Jane and the project they are working on together. Mary was threatened by Jane's budget analysis because she felt as if Jane was trying to control the situation. Whether this is true or not is beside the point and beyond the scope of analysis. If Mary spent precious time trying to figure out Jane's agenda and then responded according to what she determined it to be, think about the time she would waste. Even if she were accurate in her assessment, it would be an ineffective way for her to spend her time. She needs to focus on her performance and her role in the partnership, that is all.

In order for Mary to correctly do this step, she will need to disassociate herself from the situation. She will need to forget about the fact that she and Jane have had terrible disagreements in the past. She will put aside the fact that Jane has made insulting remarks to her about her unsuccessful projects; she will not take it personally. This step in the ERT is stellar in helping us keep our communications in check.

Taking the time, even intellectually, to assess the situation from an outside perspective is a form of therapy. It helps us to remember where we're going and how we're getting there. Moreover, it reminds us to eliminate those negative reactions that keep our interactions at a non-productive pace.

We will first demonstrate how Mary applies this situation to the scenario we have already discussed then you will complete the exercise that follows, applying it to an experience that you have already encountered. Once you realize how easy and quickly this can be applied, you will find you can take the few seconds required and automatically include this step in all of your interactions.

Mary starts by removing the emotions and listing the facts. Again, we are doing this in writing to show the process. In real life you will often find the situations that require this step don't allow anytime for pulling out paper and pen and taking notes. That's okay— this is easy enough to mentally perform, and actually should be something you work to incorporate in the back of your mind at all times.

Here are Mary's facts about the situation:

1. Jane and I have been assigned a project
2. Jane's role is to manage the budget
3. My role is to implement the plan
4. Jane has already started her work

Simply put, Mary has nothing to feel reactionary toward. By stepping outside of the situation she has discovered that, regardless of the emotional baggage, insecurities or control issues that either of them bring to the situation, this is the barebones. Jane was doing her job and now Mary has to do hers. It does not matter whether or not Jane has a hidden agenda; we are only interested in the facts right now.

Once you begin applying this you will note how short and sweet it can be, therefore, an automatic-assessment tool in virtually any communication. Let's look at one other situation and how quickly it can be applied.

Imagine you are on the phone with the electric company, sure that you have been overcharged. You know for a fact that your bill is never this high and you suspect the person who reads the meter was unable to get into the backyard so instead, an educated guess was taken at your watt usage. Your telephone conversation goes something like this:

> You: *This bill is not right, I'm telling you.*
> Clerk: *I'm sorry sir, $438 is what I show on my screen.*
> You: *But it's wrong, don't you realize what an outrageous amount that is?*
> Clerk: *I understand sir, but that's what the record indicates.*

Clearly, many of us have experienced similar situations. Losing our cool in this case would be a result of feeling as if we're not being heard or we feeling like we're being treated unfairly. Either way, reacting negatively is not going to change the fact that this clerk still shows your electric bill to be $438. A quick assessment, stepping outside of the situation, which you would do in your head at this point, might go like this:

1. The clerk can only tell me what she sees.
2. I'm sure the bill is wrong so I need to go to the next level up.

In that quick assessment, without raising your stress level or even your voice, you could simply ask the clerk to tell you how billing disputes are handled. This, she can help you with. Too many times we feel like we hit a verbal brick wall because we are not getting the responses we are looking for, when in essence, it is because we are asking the wrong questions.

The following exercise will give you an opportunity to review this step in real time application. Do not pick a situation that makes you look good; the purpose of these exercises are to help you improve your interactions and you can only do that when you allow for honest assessment. Select a situation where you were emotionally involved or challenged. It can be personal or professional. Forget the emotional components. Forget the hidden agenda that the other person or you might have had. Don't worry about competitiveness or insecurity. Instead, focus from the outside in. Look only at the facts and how they pertain to the situation. Allow yourself to be completely removed from the situation. Do not include any negative or positive remarks. Stay neutral and focused only on the facts.

Name the facts, without any reference to feeling.
1.
2.
3.
4.
5.

Now look how differently this situation appears from an outside perspective. Even if the other person did something blatantly wrong, that is beside the point and doesn't matter right now. We're not placing blame or pointing fingers, but striving to remove our emotional investment so that we can see the scene through a whole new set of eyes and operate more effectively. This is what all superior mangers, company presidents, and CEOs already know how to do; it's how they got where they are.

To increase the power of the following exercise, and gain the increased benefit, complete the following emotionally based self-assessment on one of your own experiences:

1. The reason this person upset me:

2. What I was really mad about:

3. The word that best describes my reaction:

Ask yourself these three questions each and every time you experience a communication conflict that had emotional repercussions, such as you felt cheated, threatened or angry. You will quickly begin to identify patterns. Once you better understand what kinds of communication situations tend to make you react negatively, you will be better equipped to foresee and deter them before they affect your interactions with others.

The true intent behind this book is not only to teach you how to respond effectively to other people so that you can get ahead in life, but also to provide thought-provoking ideas and exercises that make you yourself easier to communicate *with*. It is only when we take responsibility for our own role in this world that we can truly begin to evolve into compassionately successful communicators. That is the crux of effective interactions, so use these exercises wisely. Use the information to your advantage by recognizing the parts of yourself scattered throughout the pages. We all have overblown egos and insecurities that we should learn to live without.

In order to improve our lives we must improve our interactions. Our interactions and relationship with others are instrumental to our growth. Pay attention to the various roles you play and learn to incorporate these steps. The Effective Response Theory can be adopted and applied to all communication situations; from working with small children to employees, from partners to store clerks, from parents to CEO's.

In summary, when we step outside the situation, even for a brief moment, we are able to see beyond our anger and our ego and address the situation from a logical perspective. You will find yourself reaching the results you are after much more rapidly when you are able to step outside and look back in. Because we tend to fall victim to the words of others, allowing their ego-based remarks to impact our egos and insecurities, here is the fail-proof solution to stop you in your tracks:

Ask Yourself......How Does This Affect My Life?

The way you pose the question can vary to fit each situation. Let's look at an example. Say you are sitting at your desk having a conversation with the office accountant who informs you that he was voted most popular in his senior year of high school. You know this to be untrue. Say you know someone he went to high school with who has verified for you that his pocket protector days go way back beyond high school. This kind of situation is so common in everyday conversation. Someone says something that you feel certain they are wrong about. In many instances, if not most, what the other guy is saying is simply something that makes him or her feel bigger and better in your eyes...so take it as a compliment. Too many of us are bound and determined to "prove" somebody wrong, and nothing gets the adrenaline flowing like a challenge of rightness.

In the case of the accountant above, you have to ask yourself the qualifying question, or a form of it. How does this affect my life? Does it matter to me one iota that this guy is living in fairytale town and thinks he was popular? Does it affect anything at all in the scheme of things?

When the answer is no, you should drop the issue. If someone fabricates the truth or simply makes a mistaken remark, unless it has a true impact on something (and your own ego doesn't count) then simply learn to let it slide. Not only will you greatly reduce your own level of stress, you'll be taking great strides to help someone do what we all try and do, feel important.

If you were to tell the accountant that you knew for a fact that he was a nerd in high school, never even coming close to winning any "most popular person" award, what exactly do you think you would accomplish? Would proving him wrong, making him feel bad, just to show him and the world that you had a leg up, really be worth it? Highly unlikely. The way you can tell if it's simply your own ego at the wheel is to consider whether or not the situation would make a big difference in somebody's life.

In other words, if the accountant had a thousand dollar bet with you that he was voted most popular in high school (shame on you for betting), then you're probably going to feel compelled to prove your point. On the same note, if someone is lying about something that is causing someone else pain, the truth can be worth tracking down.

There are as many situations as there are people, and sometimes the lines will blur. The trick, however, in determining the right direction to take is by asking the qualifying question, "How does this affect my life?" Actually, there are a number of questions you might apply that result in precisely the same thing:

Will this hurt anyone?

Will this change the world?

Will this make a difference in my life tomorrow?

Is anyone going to go to war over this?

Would the newspaper be reporting this?

Essentially, you've got to ask whatever question it is that will help you differentiate between your morals and your ego. Often times we can fool ourselves into thinking it's our high moral standards that have us standing up to the opposition, putting them in their place. For instance, if you are witnessing two people at the office disagree about a company policy, and you know the guy on the left is right, are you speaking up and pulling out your policy manual because you think he can't speak and think for him self, or is this a crack shot at fueling your own ego? Usually, it's the latter.

You have to ask yourself, when these two employees are disagreeing about the company policy, does it really affect your life? Is it really important enough for you to let your ego get all dressed up and head for town? Not likely.

Learning to let go is hard. It takes a certain amount of trust to believe that people who fabricate will eventually be put in their place, but let it be of their own accord, not your gallant efforts to save the day. Furthermore, understand that you have been just as guilty of publicly massaging your ego; it's just that now you know how inappropriate and ineffective it really is. People like to feel important, so let them.

Chapter Ten
PUT ON YOUR WALKIN' SHOES

HOW many times have we heard the expression, "Walk a mile in his shoes?" That's what this step of ERT focuses on. Because we are creatures of habit, often consumed with our own vested interest in any given situation, it can only do us good to remember that the other person is equally self-consumed. We are each the star in our own life story. It is only when we consider the other person's stake in the game that we can genuinely communicate. Nothing will bring you closer to improved interactions than your ability to walk in the other person's shoes, wear their hat, or to get a glimpse of life through their looking-glasses. So slip on somebody else's shoes, and start walking.

In Dale Carnegie's best-selling book, *How to Win Friends and Influence People,* Practice Number Eight is, "Try to honestly see things from the other person's point of view." Defined, this is exactly the same thing as walking in the other person's shoes. It is only when we see the world from another's perspective that we are looking at the same sunset. A good analogy of changing views for many people is this: Most of us, at some time or another, have been seated in an audience. How different does that view become from up on the stage? Same room, same audience, different perspective. It's an entirely new look at the same thing and it can make all the difference in the world. Another example is a traffic accident. How many witnesses have different or varying stories? Something as simple as a fender bender might have several supporting stories, yet only one is completely accurate. Does that mean people are intentionally telling mistruths? Not necessarily. Simply put, people see what they *think* they see, even if it's slightly off. Understanding this, that everyone is entitled to their own perspective, is helpful in seeing things from a different vantage point.

Walking in the other person's shoes is all about empathy. It's about assuming a new view out of respect for others. In the previous chapter, we took a look at the situation by stripping away our emotional baggage and making a logical assessment. In this step we allow for the emotional baggage, only it's theirs, not ours. It is entirely possible to assess your actions without including your own emotions, yet allowing for the emotions of others. It keeps you humble and makes you human. People respond best to people who seem to care. When you take the time to see the good intentions of others, you can't help but be a better communicator.

Walking in the other person's shoes means looking at the situation through her eyes, empathizing with her role, and acknowledging that you don't necessarily know more than she does. There is usually at least two sides to every story, yet we are continuously trained to operate only from the side we see best (which inevitably is the side that we benefit most). When we perfect this skill of empathy, it will be reflected in all of our interactions. People will not only enjoy our company, but they will be eager to assist in whatever way they can. This is the part of the Effective Communication Theory where we put on their shoes and take a little walk.

Looking at a situation through someone else's eyes means you have to eliminate your own ego and insecurities, while keeping theirs in tact. For instance, you need to forget that you were threatened by the way your boss talked to you and realize that he must have been threatened himself to use the tone he did. This is not always an easy thing to do. We already have acknowledged that reacting negatively is almost instinctual. If someone yells, we yell back, if someone gives us the cold shoulder, maybe we do the same. This step of the theory takes you from opponent to friend.

Remember that everyone has stress, late bills, fights with their honey, bosses who demand too much and not enough hours in the day. This being the case, it is easy to see why we often become impatient and snappy. The irony though is that we can instantly understand and accept our own errors, but we are hard pressed to do so with others. While we're reacting negatively to the paperboy because he's ten minutes late, we're not considering his own reaction for being ten minutes late.

We fail to see the forest for the trees. All we can think about is that our newspaper was delivered ten minutes late. Those are ten minutes we would peruse the stock section, read our horoscope, and breeze through the comics before heading off to work. Of course we are irritated, but consider this: the paperboy is going to have numerous people who are potentially and equally irritated with him. He probably is afraid that some of his customers might call the paper and complain. Because we are so busy being mad or feeling cheated, we're not considering the whole situation. Any situation, of course, is relative. For example, if your paperboy is always late, then perhaps there is a problem and he *should* be replaced. More often than not though, we are quick to point out the errors of others, giving little consideration to those that we have made ourselves.

This is not to state that you shouldn't, at times, complain, stand your ground, or ask to speak to the next person in charge. It is, however, intended to serve as a guide that helps you realize that other people have other problems and just like you are the star of your own universe, they are the star of theirs.

In the national bestseller, *Getting To Yes,* authors Roger Fisher and William Ury advise readers how to successfully win at corporate negotiations. Even here, their direction correctly assigns value to empathic understanding, "Don't attack their position, look behind it. When the other side sets forth their position, neither reject it nor accept it. Treat it as one possible option. Look for the interests behind it, seek out the principles which it reflects, and think about ways to improve it."

The person who you are interacting with has an equally vested interest that is no less or no more valid than your own. Once you respect and operate from that understanding, you will have a much clearer view of the overall situation. By grasping this concept and learning to employ the strategy of empathy in your interactions, you will be a much better communicator (and the paperboy will love you).

It doesn't mean that you have to take any great strides or make any grand efforts that truly go against your grain. Most of the time, simply considering how the other person might be seeing things is enough. Maybe it won't change anything you say or do, but it will give you a perspective that you didn't have before, and chances are the other person will notice it.

Another good scenario is when we are at a very busy store or establishment and we are growing impatient. There is a huge line and the store staff is obviously short-handed. How many people are standing in line, rolling their eyes, irritated, maybe even complaining out loud? This is not to say that waiting in a long line is not frustrating. However, what happens when you walk in the clerk's shoes? She's got the pressure of performing quickly, knowing that all of these people are growing increasingly hostile. She's so overly conscientious about making mistakes that she makes many, only slowing her down more and making the line of people grow angrier.

Consider this: You are a parent and your first year college student comes home simply exasperated. As a parent, you are concerned and supportive.

"What happened today?"

"First day at work, wasn't so easy."

"What happened?"

"Oh, one of the other girls didn't show up, the line got really long, and everyone got mad at me. I made a bunch of mistakes and someone even complained to the manager."

Do you see how different you feel about the same scenario of waiting in a long line when you take the time to realize the fact that the person behind the counter is no different, than say, your own kid? Kind of softens your heart, doesn't it? Regardless of how smart us humans tend to get, we often fall way behind in our ability to view situations from different perspectives.

This is no insinuation of whether or not the girl behind the counter could have done things differently; that's anybody's guess. We're talking here about perceptions and how they vary tremendously with different people. Surely, even her boss has a different perspective, and if you asked all of the people in line what they were thinking, you'd get a sprinkling of different responses as well. The point is that it is not our place or our challenge to determine the correctness of a situation, but rather to view the situation empathetically through the other party's eyes. Walk in his shoes before you react and your response will be much more effective.

What might happen if every person in that line walked in the store clerk's shoes? What if they all stopped and remembered a time that they were in a similar situation? A time when they didn't have control, had lots of pressure, and people were standing by with critical looks on their faces? The answer is obvious; the people in line would become more patient and empathetic, the store clerk would feel more at ease and ultimately increase her cash registering speed. By seeing things a different way we are in a much better position to produce more positive results.

We all play different roles in the various communication we enter. The common problem is that we assume the way *we* feel is correct. We judge others as if we are somehow superior. We are not. We assume that the other person is playing by the same rules that we ourselves have imposed when this is seldom the case. It is only when we walk in their shoes that we see the situation in a fair light. Constantly consumed with our own point of view, we often overlook the fact that those we are interacting with come with a perspective that might be very different from our own. When we dare to put our egos and insecurities aside we are usually surprised that other people have ideas, fears, and motivations every bit as valid as our own. It is by no coincidence that we are easy to blame others for things we might be just as guilty of ourselves.

Consider dishonesty in a politician. While we are certainly not condoning dishonesty of any sort, it is interesting to debate the public reaction. How many people who criticize dishonesty in the White House have not also been guilty of lying or immoral acts they too would deny? Again, this is not to endorse or promote dishonesty, but rather to help you understand how differently we view the same situation from a different perspective.

If you were discovered cheating on your tax returns, chances are you would have a reason, a justification of sorts. Regardless though, you cheated and you got caught. Is this something you would want publicized throughout your place of employment? Would you write letters to all of your distant relatives and tell them about your unethical behavior? Send out a press release? Chances are the answer is no.

You might argue and say a politician has a professional and moral obligation to be honest and hold no secrets from his public, and that is fine. The point is that we are usually quick to dissect others when we are often made up of the same fiber. It is easy to see when someone else has done wrong, yet when it is us who has erred, we prefer to overlook it. We sweep it under the carpet and hope it goes away

When you learn to walk in the other person's shoes you learn to see things from his point of view. The best way to see another point of view is to imagine you were in the same situation as the other guy and then think about how you might feel.

One of the tricks of learning to empathize comes with understanding process. Understanding process does not work with all interactions. For example, you might be challenged to use this technique at the drive-thru window of your favorite fast food place when the clerk forgot your fries. However, understanding the process that people go through can be applied to many aspects of your professional and personal life.

There are processes for dozens of the events we all experience. From the death of a loved one; to childbirth; to dieting; to purchasing decisions, there is often a standard process that prevails. If you are in sales, this component of empathy will be your strongest selling point. "Process" simply refers to the general stages the person immersed in the situation will go through. For example, psychologists note that the process we go through when we lose someone we love usually includes the stages of shock, denial, guilt, and grief. When you understand the stage of any given process a person is going through, you are in a better position to understand how they feel. Another example would be falling in love. A person will be in a much different state of mind (or stage of process) when they first start dating the person of their dreams as opposed, say, to when they find out that person has been having an affair. All of life is filled with processes of one kind or another.

Even life itself is a process. A person who is just getting married, for example, is in a different stage than a person getting ready to retire. Both are at the threshold of a new beginning. Some might say one is starting something and one is ending something, but that would be untrue. They are both starting something new (not having to work anymore and committing to another person. And they are both ending something (a career and bachelorhood). Yet these are entirely new starts and ending. The mindsets and emotional stages will be completely different too. They have different agendas. Being aware of these differences and how they might color the individuals' perceptions, opinions, and feelings, is helpful toward productive interactions. In some cases, it is critical to effective communications.

Let's look at the basic concept of buying a car. Generally speaking, and without considering the individual in question, a car salesperson might assess that there are several stages a person goes through when buying a car. For example, there is one stage that the salesperson calls "the fear stage." Maybe the fear stage is after the customer has test-driven the car, settled on a price, and sat down for financing terms. All of a sudden, the fear hits him. It's occurred to him that he will be committing to a huge monthly payment that might cut deeply into his other goal of buying a new house.

The wise salesman or woman will recognize this stage and respond to it directly and effectively. Not understanding this stage of the buying process, the salesperson could easily lose the customer and never know why. When a person is operating from a place of fear, logical argument will hold little ground. A person feeling fearful needs reassurance. In order for the salesperson to understand this, he would have to be able to recognize the fear in the customer and walk in his shoes right down that same scary path. This is an area that the most effective salespeople excel in.

Regardless of your business, if you operate in an arena where there is any kind of "standardized" processes, you should become proficient at recognizing and responding to them. Even in your personal life, you will note that your spouse, parents, children, and next door neighbors go through various processes throughout their lives. Processes simply represent the stage we are experiencing at any given time. The stage we are in often lends some insight to the way we are feeling. When we understand how someone feels, we are that much closer to walking in his shoes.

Another example someone once shared involved mothers who were going back to work after having babies. The day care worker, in this instance, explained that mothers returning to work go through a series of stages as it relates to leaving their child in day care. The first stage might be depression or guilt. The smart daycare worker will already know this and be much more effective in her communications with the mother based on this awareness. The mothers then, respond to the empathy and are better able to adjust to leaving their children when they go back to work.

In most offices, there are generally processes of some sort or another. Businesses run on systems and systems usually mean processes. Think now of some of the processes in your own life, whether personal or professional, that might give you a better understanding as to what someone else is experiencing. By being aware of the processes that are already in place, you have taken a gigantic step toward empathizing with the person who is experiencing the process. People respond to empathy.

Think for example, of a time when you were arguing your point in the board- room. Maybe one other person supported you, stood up in your favor and agreed with what you said. Didn't you think that person was smart? Didn't that person automatically earn a place on your holiday shopping list? This is how other people will feel about you if you take the time to understand how they might be seeing things and then respond accordingly.

Customer service surveys and studies have indicated that the majority of customers who call and complain merely want to be heard. Empathized with. Consider the two following examples and conclude which one would be more effective.

Example One:
Customer Service: *No Sir, we can't refund your money.*
Customer: *But it broke, the stupid thing broke after only six months!*
Customer Service: *I'm sorry sir. The unit only has a 30-day warranty.*
Customer: *I need a new one and I don't want to pay for it!*

Example Two:
Customer Service: *No Sir, we can't refund your money, but I understand how you must feel.*

Customer: *But it broke, the stupid thing broke after only six months!*

Customer Service: *That must be very frustrating for you, how did it break?*

****

Presumably the customer won't get the money back in either scenario, however, in the second example, chances are that the customer will buy a new one, or at the very least, feel somehow more consoled and less frustrated than with the first interaction. And at any rate, will be less likely to make derogatory remarks about the company as a whole. The customer service clerk used empathy. When you walk in the other person's shoes, it's easy to empathize. It's simply a matter of focusing on someone else's pain for a moment, instead of your own. Considering the other person in your communication efforts will take you much farther than any amount of work you could do on your speech or delivery. When you empathize, you put your heart into the interaction. In the art of empathy it can often help to summarize the presumed position of the other party. This not only verifies for them that you are stepping outside of your own realm, trying to look at things from their perspective, but it gives them the chance to think about and get in better touch with how they are feeling. Then, if your assumption is wrong, it can easily be corrected.

Example:

You: *I'm sorry I didn't get that report to you on time. It must have made you mad.*

Co-worker: *No, actually it kind of hurt my feelings that you might have forgotten about me.*

This is a prime example of how easily and often we miscalculate another person's point of view. By making the effort and taking the time to empathize, we've shown the other person our genuine interest in the interaction. Then, if we've misjudged the situation, the other person is more likely to clear things up, giving us a better understanding as to how she really feel, since we cared enough to comment. Certainly we would respond and communicate differently to someone who was angry with us versus someone who was feeling wounded because of us.

The last component for walking in their shoes is to never assume. Regardless of what kind of legend you might be in your own mind, you only know what you know and you don't know everything.

Not assuming means you give the other person a chance to explain. It means you are empathetic in regard to not jumping the gun about something you might know nothing about. An example to keep in mind will serve to remind you of this simple but poignant fact.

A printer had promised Terry he would have her big printing project done by Monday. Terry and the printer had done a few projects together before but this one was a high priority and meant a lot to Terry's career. The printer called Terry on Thursday afternoon and told her things were right on schedule and that to ensure the project was delivered first thing Monday morning, he was going to work Friday night and Saturday until the job was done. Terry felt assured the project would be completed in a timely manner.

Monday morning at 7:55 the printer called and told Terry the job was not ready. He apologized, and told her he knew how important it was. He said he could have it done by Wednesday. Terry was outraged. She lost her cool and blew up at the printer.

Not once did she stop to empathize, to consider that there could be a reason for the hold up. It was only a week later that she learned the Friday night the printer had planned to work on the project, his wife was killed in an automobile accident.

You don't know everything and when you react as if you do, you are more likely to say and do things that take you farther from your goals and make you look bad to other people. Of course Terry felt awful and eventually apologized, but she was too embarrassed to ever do business with that particular printer again. She had failed to give him the benefit of the doubt. Find out what's going on before you react. Empathizing is an appropriate place to start. You can let someone know you are deeply disturbed, put off, or disappointed in their actions or their words, but start by finding out why the thing occurred in the first place; it may change everything.

It's an undeniable fact that we often get what we expect. When you expect that people are inherently good, it is no coincidence that the majority of people you come across are just that. Conversely, if you expect that people are generally worthless, you're going to find that to be true as well. When you expect people are generally good and then act in accordance with that assumption, it will be easier to remember to apply empathy in you interactions. Don't ever assume that you know everything all of the time. People experience things that you may be unaware of, and many times there are valid reasons for things that happen. When you jump to conclusions without any kind of empathy or understanding, you are setting yourself up for disaster.

To better remind you to empathize, complete the exercises that follow.

Situation:

A co-worker has left early without leaving the report she promised she would deliver. Even though your first reaction is anger, list a few things that could have warranted (not caused) this occurrence.

1._____

2._____

3._____

How can you address this issue with her in a manner that allows for explanation?

Situation:

You are settling an insurance claim. Your role as underwriter is to interview the claimants, who, in this case, lost their home to fire. The woman is being difficult. Put yourself in her shoes and explain how you might be more effective:

_____
_____
_____
_____
_____

Name a recent experience where your empathy would have helped the interaction:

_____
_____

If you walked in the other person's shoes, what might have you of seen?

_____

Chapter Eleven
ASK FOR AN ANSWER

THE only way we can ever learn what we need to know is by asking questions. If you are a waitress in a café and you don't ask the customer what he wants to eat, instead just bring him what you think he'd like to have, chances are your tip won't be very big. Questions are our perfect opportunity to interact more efficiently.

Asking questions is an integral part of the Effective Response Theory. It is only through inquiry we can find out, directly from the person we are communicating with, what it is we need to know in order to make the interaction more productive. Asking smart questions is the key. We will discuss the different kinds of questions you can ask, how you can help shift thinking with the proper questions, and how you can let people sell themselves on your ideas. All of this is done with smart questions.

Our interactions with others are organic. They are living growing things that must be nurtured to expansion. Asking questions is the easiest way to foster an interaction that has positive results. In the Book, *The 7 Powers of Questions,* Dorothy Leeds tells us that wisely worded questions can help shift the conversation into the most desirable direction. "You can use questions to help other people shift their focus in just about any situation: when you are trying to solve personal problems, when you are speaking with your children, when you are trying to make a sale, or when you are coaching an employee."

Let's put this into practice and see how it works. In this example, a manager, who is talking to an employee that is upset because a co-worker has made some inappropriate remarks, has the task of investigating the validity of the claim, determining if it needs to escalate to HR, and getting her otherwise productive employee back on track.

The right questions can take the employee from a place of self-centered frustration to a more productive role. Instead of just identifying and complaining about the co-worker, she can be guided into becoming a part of the solution.

Here are some examples the smart manager might pose to his complaining employee:

- ❑ Why do you think this is happening?
- ❑ How do you think we should handle it?
- ❑ What could we say to her to make her stop?
- ❑ Do you think she's aware of what she's saying?
- ❑ Have you mentioned how you feel?
- ❑ Have you noticed her acting this way with anyone else?
- ❑ Do you think it would help if I talked with her?
- ❑ Should we call her in now?

Notice that the list of questions presents a very team-oriented approach to problem solving. Think of how much more effective the questions above are then the more reactionary questions that many managers might ask under the same circumstances. A list of common questions for the same scenario might be: how did you provoke this? Should I report it to HR? Did you insult her somehow? Have you discussed this with her? Can't you manage to get along? Isn't this something that can be overlooked? Clearly, these questions aren't nearly as likely to promote a productive outcome or foster trust and growth.

Instead, the second set of questions would tend to make the employee wish she had never come forward. While some managers might seem satisfied with the idea of employees not coming forward, consider the consequences. Low moral and unhappy employees will always and inevitably affect production.

Whether it is complaints, ideas, or comments, employees need to be prompted with questions that work. Even in your personal life, the same rules apply. If you don't believe this, try having a conversation with a child who has just gotten into trouble and doesn't want to talk about it. A child's common response to the wrong kind of question is, "I don't know." What they are really saying is, "You are not asking me a question that gives me the opportunity to express the point I am trying to make," but "I don't know" is just the way it comes out.

The good news in the book, *More Power To You*, the authors inform us that women traditionally have been shown to ask up to three times as many questions as their male counterparts. A lifetime of needing to initiate conversations with non-communicative fathers, husbands, and sons, has turned us in to a gender that knows how to ask what she wants to know! Asking gets us where we need to go and more.

The right questions allow us to shift the other person's thinking in a direction that brings us closer to our goals and helps them find a solution to the problem or the issue at hand.

People are only too glad to answer your questions, especially when it concerns them. Remember what we said earlier, people are the stars of their own show; they appreciate an interested audience. Asking questions about what the other person thinks, feels, and knows is a sure way to win his respect and appreciation. It doesn't matter if you're asking a child to tell you how he won the spelling bee or a co-worker to recount the details of her cruise. People love to answer questions about themselves.

Remember to ask the kinds of questions that count; the ones that take you where you'd like to go with regards to a productive interaction. This is more than simply being the life of the party. While learning to speak in an affable manner is undoubtedly an excellent skill to develop, our intent is to learn to use our communication skills in a way that produces the results we're after; being a great conversationalist is a by product of it all. Good questions make us better speakers.

Beyond asking questions for more productive interactions in general, consider asking questions as a means of gathering information about people you know. The more you know about someone, the better you will be at communicating with him or her. This is true because when you are more aware of someone's thinking process, the role they play in any given situation, and the way they might be feeling, you are that much better equipped to interact optimally.

Consider how the best salespeople always know how many kids you have, where you went on vacation, and what your favorite kind of candy is. Smart data collection is an integral part of top-producing sales. And, all of this information you gather will be conducive to supporting your overall efforts at improved interactions.

Ask people about their likes and dislikes, their passions and their strengths. Any effective communicator understands that the better we understand others, the better we understand ourselves, and that information always makes us more effective in our purposes.

Before we begin exploring the kinds of questions you should ask, let's take a moment to discuss self-questioning techniques. As suggested in the book, *7 Powers of Questions,* "This self-questioning is essential to our growth, because it helps us examine ourselves. Self-questioning cannot only help us determine our successes and our failures, but it can help us understand the reasons behind those outcomes."

We already noted earlier that the primary question you will want to keep in your mind during any kind of interaction is: "Is this taking me closer to my goals?" And clearly, that is probably the most important question any of us can ask ourselves prior to ever opening our mouths. Let us consider the kind of self-questions that might lend us a better sense of understanding toward the kind of communicators we really are.

At the beginning we talked about how many of our poor interactions result from our negative reactions as opposed to effective responses. By asking questions as they occur, or even in retrospect, we are much more likely to understand, hence take control of those weaknesses in our communication skills. Consider a conversation that takes place between two store clerks who are setting up a window display. The first clerk is dressing the mannequins and the second clerk is decorating the backdrop. The first clerk tells the second clerk her idea, and the second clerk disagrees. The conversation might go something like this:

> Clerk one: *I think a dark green background would really pull the colors of this suit.*

Clerk two: *Yes, but this is a spring window, so lavender is more appropriate.*

Clerk one: *We're tying to be different, non-traditional. Spring can be any color we say it is.*

Neither clerk is wrong. Both clerks have ownership over a particular portion of the task that they are responsible for. So how could self-questioning help resolve their disagreement? In situations that are not life changing there is nothing wrong with compromise. This does not mean you need to roll over and give in every time you experience a difference of opinion. For this scenario, let's make Clerk two the hero and the one who decides to ask self-questions.

1. Is a dark green window going to have any negative impact on anything beyond my ego?
2. Am I just being hardheaded because I want my way?
3. Will less people be drawn to the window because it isn't my idea of traditional?
4. Is there any chance of compromise?
5. Will the world fall apart if there isn't a lavender background?
6. Are there other great clothes that would match the green background?

While this list of questions could be longer, it can often be much shorter. The point is, whenever any kind of disagreement surfaces, no matter how seemingly large or small, you have to question your intent. You have to ask yourself whether the world will stop spinning if you do not get your way and whether there is a valid, legitimate reason why your way is better. If you respond in a manner that says compromise is possible, not only will you avoid or curb a negative reaction in the other party, you will soon become their ally:

Clerk two: Okay, tell you what, I'll pick out some different outfits that match your dark green backdrop. How about next month, we go with the traditional pastels.

Clerk one: You've got yourself a deal! Thanks.

You have to ask yourself, anytime you are about to take on a battle, is it really worth the time, trouble, and effort? If not, you are often better off reserving your energy for communications that have more significant value in your life. So asking the kinds of self-questions that help us immediately resolve the issue or interaction at hand is one way to become more effective. Additionally, there are questions we can ask ourselves that help us understand more deeply *why* we feel the need to react negatively in certain situations.

For example, during our discussion on negative reactions, we talked about the way our ego and our insecurities tend to shade our communication skills. When certain things set our triggers off, we might react wildly, leaving our sanity behind us. These are prime times to question ourselves about our motives.

For instance, if you were Clerk One in the scenario above and you felt your heartbeat increase, your stress level rise, and your knees start to shake, then quite clearly the communication has hit a trigger that warrants further exploration. This is the time to ask yourself pointed questions that might better enable you to understand, hence improve, your interaction triggers.

> What about that bothers me?
> Am I taking this too personally?
> Why do I need to be in charge?
> Do I feel like she's challenging me?
> What can I learn from this?
> What in my past does this remind me of?

The list might be endless, or, you might not even be able to think of one question if you are in the middle of a physical and emotional reaction. However, because self-questions are truly vital for your continued advancement, take advantage of every opportunity to understand yourself better. There are two exercises that follow. Each asks you to name a situation that might cause a reaction. You will also be prompted to ask some of your own questions. Use one of these for a professional interaction and the other for a personal one.

This is only scratching the surface, however, you are that much closer and that much more aware of the kinds of things that make you tick. As you communicate, pay attention to those feelings that arise and tend to make you feel panicked and compelled to react. Try and remember at that crucial point to ask yourself what is it that has you feeling so threatened. Identifying the culprit is the first step in eliminating it.

Exercise:

Think of a work-related situation that made you feel reactionary. It doesn't matter whether or not you bit your tongue or exploded. That is beside the point. Think the situation though and describe it below, then answer the questions:

Situation:_____

_____

_____

_____

_____

What was it specifically that bothered you about this situation?

_____

_____

_____

Why?

_____

_____

_____

How did this situation threaten you?

_____

_____

_____

_____

Now ask yourself more feeling-finding questions that will help you gain a better understanding as to why you wanted to react the way you did. Then answer them.

_____

_____

_____

_____

Exercise:

Think of a personal situation that made you want to react. It doesn't matter whether or not you bit your tongue or exploded. That is beside the point. Think of the situation and describe it below, then answer the questions:

Situation:_____

_____

_____

_____

What was it specifically that bothered you about this situation?

_____

_____

_____

Why?

_____

_____

How did this situation threaten you?

_____

_____

_____

Now ask yourself more feeling-finding questions that will help you gain a better understanding as to why you wanted to react the way you did. Then answer them.

_____

_____

_____

_____

_____

_____

There are many modes of modern-day therapy that can help us delve head first into those issues of our past that tend to cause us problems and stand in the very way of our productivity. It is a mistake to think that if you suffered any kind of trauma in the past that it won't inadvertently and "un-invitedly" pop up when you least expect it. Worse yet, some of the things that impact us most severely might not even be qualified as real trauma.

For example, something as simple as your birthing order might affect your outlook on life. Say you were the middle child, always feeling overlooked and out of place. There surely could be situations that arise in your adult life that trigger those old forgotten feelings of inadequacy. Those feelings that get triggered can make effective communications often times impossible.

Without delving too deeply into our psychological background and make-up, understand the obvious. If there are parts of your past that remain unhealed or unprocessed, issues that you have kept covered up and hidden, you will have a hard time being the kind of communicator that makes a difference. The good news is that there are currently some very effective (and quick) therapy techniques that can have you in and out and feeling better in no time. If this sounds like something you are interested in, check with a mental health professional that specializes in an area of your particular interests or needs. The stigma of only weak or "crazy" people needing therapy has long been replaced with the realization that the better condition we are in mentally and emotionally, the more mountains we can climb. We are exceedingly more productive when we strive to understand our emotions and motivations and take charge of our direction.

Recognizing our triggers is the first step in repairing them. Remember the Big Truth: *You can't change anything but yourself.* Just because you tend to react emotionally whenever someone else points their index finger (because it reminds you of your wicked stepmother), doesn't mean you can go around the world warning folks to keep their hands in their pockets; it's your responsibility to learn to deal with the triggers, the people and the situations that send you off the deep end. At the very least, learn to carry a lifejacket.

There have been several thought-provoking books written on the art of dealing with difficult people or people you dislike. The main problem with these kinds of books is that they tend to try and categorize people into certain groups. We've already noted that there are flaws in this way of thinking. However, if you expand and pursue your self-investigation into trigger points, you can learn some very interesting things about yourself as it relates to the people, or types of people, that are most difficult for you to deal with.

It is by no coincidence that someone you cannot stand seems to get along well with other people you know. This is true in both your personal and professional life. You ask yourself how someone who is so obnoxious can possibly be liked by _____(fill in the blank). It's hard to understand how someone that you see as being clearly despicable can be liked by others. Part of our overall effort to interact well with other people is for us to learn effective ways to interact with ourselves. The "problems" we sometimes see in others, are really nothing more than a reflection of the shortcomings we see in ourselves. The world is a mirror...what do you see?

This isn't always such an easy concept to grasp, so let's take a closer look. The parts we despise in others are parts of ourselves we either dislike, or are not in touch with. This works in a couple of different ways. The most common way is this: Say you abhor selfish people. Just being around someone who is a tightwad makes your skin crawl. Now ask yourself, what is it about your own selfishness that you need to deal with?

The world and the people in it are a direct reflection of who we each are. The world really is a mirror, and if you look closely and pay attention, you will undoubtedly catch your own reflection. The parts of our own personalities that come up short are the very traits that will bother us in those around us. This is exactly why Joe may drive you bonkers but not bother your friend Amy at all. Joe might be really outgoing— people might love him— but he sends you right over the edge. Is Joe's obnoxious outgoing personality so annoying because your own outgoingness is hindered or hidden and you resent seeing it in Joe? Or maybe, you see that loud side of yourself and don't feel comfortable with the possibility of other people seeing you in the same light you see Joe.

If it bothers you deeply that a co-worker gossips, is there a gossiping part of you that you refuse to get in touch with?

Take a moment now and make a list of those few people you have known in your lifetime who really sent you reeling, really drove you mad. There probably isn't more than a handful, so the list shouldn't be too long. It doesn't have to be someone you literally hate, hopefully no such list of that nature exists, but rather, those people you've known who have caused you to react negatively. Those people who have tested your sanity and your patience. Perhaps it's a previous boss, an ex-partner, the landlord, or your best friend's husband. It might be the office manager or a professor you had in college. Write it down. This exercise is highly effective in discovering things about yourself you might not otherwise be aware of (it might not be so fun at first to find faults in yourself, but once you spot them, they're easier to eliminate and work through).

1.

2.

3.

4.

5.

After you've written your list, under each person's name, write a couple of specific reasons that the person bothered you. These reasons should not be general, such as, "She had a big ego," but more specific. For example, "She needed constant reassurance that her clothing looked good." Do this for each person. You might need more paper, but don't skip this step. Putting something down like, "He fired me," is specific in nature, but not in cause. There had to be some kind of background that transpired well before the termination. Remember, these are people who really drove you batty and it generally requires a history of repetitive events or situations, not a one-time occurrence.

Now that you have a list of those people you've tended to react to (or wanted to) in the past, and you have listed specific things that bothered you about them, it's time to look at yourself. For each item you selected, think about what you see in yourself. Don't say you don't see anything because if it were not something that had an emotional affect, you'd never have noted it in the first place. For example, if you noted one thing that drove you crazy about a woman you worked with who always needed confirmation that she was attractive, what does that mean for you?

Perhaps you would like confirmation that you are attractive, but are too afraid to ask. Or, maybe you felt competitive. Give it some thought and write it down. If you do this exercise now and anytime someone enters your life that drives you crazy, it will help you come to terms with what characteristic it is you might need to address in yourself.

The earth doesn't spin on some ambiguous schedule; there is rhyme and reason for just about everything that happens on this planet, the whole universe for that matter. To that end, isn't it likely that certain people come into your life on purpose, or for a purpose? Perhaps these are people who are intended to show you parts of yourself that you may not want to see or deal with. We all have parts that need to grow or heal. Remember always, *like attracts like.*

Understanding that we are mirrors for the rest of the world, and looking at the kinds of people we interact with on a regular basis, can lend great insight as to who we are and what *we* are reflecting for the rest of the world to see. Never underestimate the things you can learn about your self simply by asking the right questions and then answering them honestly.

It's been said before that objections are simply unanswered questions. Think about this for a moment. If you are explaining a program to your boss who doesn't seem to be responsive to the idea, perhaps he is wondering, how will this help me? Or, what will this mean to the bottom line? These are likely questions instead of objections. Help yourself by responding to these unasked inquires.

Using a sales example once more, consider a person getting ready to put down a deposit on a washer and dryer. The person might object to the price by stating that last year the set was $90 cheaper. While this statement sounds and feels just like an objection, it can easily be turned into a question, and the astute salesperson will see it as such. The potential customer is really asking one or all of the following questions:

"Why is it more expensive this year?"
"Are there any sales coming up?"
"Can you negotiate on this price?"
"Can I find it somewhere else cheaper?"
"Will it go up again next year?"
"Will I be happy with this investment?"

By viewing objections as questions in disguise and then responding effectively to the objections as if you are providing answers to unasked questions, you will go much farther than simply counter-attacking the objections. Now let's look at the different kinds of questions you will be asking people.

Traditionally speaking, there are open-ended questions and closed-ended questions. Each kind of question has a time and place and each can be effective in taking the communication in the direction you would like it to go.

Open-ended questions are preferred in most instances because they allow the respondent to elaborate his or her point. More importantly, they require the respondent to use his or her own words and descriptions. This can be very helpful when you are attempting to understand the other person's motivation and level of interest. Open-ended questions, such as, why, how, where, and what, cause the respondent to provide more than just a simple "yes" or "no" answer.

If you are trying to understand why a co-worker let you down, a child got home late, a boss is letting you go, open-ended questions will be the most effective. The intent of open-ended questions is to give you a deeper insight into the interaction. Use these question types to better understand the situation and the person you are communicating with.

Closed-ended questions have a place as well. "Did you take the cookie out of the cookie jar?" is a pretty basic question that asks exactly what you want to know. Yes or no questions are closed-ended, but so are multiple-choice questions. Many wise communicators, especially sales people, learn how to use the option technique with highly effective results. "Would you prefer the car in blue or silver?" "Would you like to sign the contract here or inside?"

Whether it is intended for persuasive purposes or as part of a fact-finding mission, closed-end questions definitely have their role in effective communications. Understanding the differences between question types is vital. Remember that open-ended questions give unlimited room for reply, whereas, closed-ended questions restrict the anticipated response. Even closed-ended questions can lead to open-ended questions. Observe the following:

Susan: *Do you like the opera?* (this is a closed-ended question, calling for a yes or no answer)

Carol: *Yes*

Susan: *What is your favorite part?* (this is an open-ended question)

Here, Susan started her communication with Carol by asking a closed-ended question. She knew before she started a conversational topic that she needed to do some fact-finding. She asked a closed-ended question to which Carol responded affirmatively, and so Susan can continue to improve the quality of the communication by going forward with an open-ended question, "What is your favorite part?"

Learn to work all kinds of questions into your communications as a matter of course. The more questions you ask, the greater the opportunity for you to learn. The more you learn and understand about yourself and the people you are communicating with, the farther you will go in this old world.

Chapter Twelve
DID YOU HEAR THAT?

WE have two ears and one mouth, yet aren't we more efficient at operating the middle unit? There have literally been hundreds of book written on the art of listening. The Effective Response Theory recognizes the act of listening as instrumental to productive interactions.

You cannot possibly respond effectively if you have not heard what has been said. Sometimes, it is not only words we must be listening to, but that which also goes unspoken. In this section, we will review the art of listening as it applies to the Theory. We will discuss how listening helps us to become better communicators. We will also consider listening to more than just the words that are being uttered. This includes body language, unspoken motivations or hearing with your heart, and finally, the art of repeating what you've heard in the form of feedback.

People enjoy being listened to, but more accurately, they like being heard. In order to reach the highest possible standard of effective communications you will need to become an expert listener. An expert listener is someone who hears what is being said as well as what is not necessarily being said. It is a person who is able to repeat back what they've heard for clarification and accuracy. Not everyone knows how to listen.

The reason we tend to make lousy listeners is because we are much more amused with our own anecdotes than we are with those of others. As we pointed out earlier, it is not uncommon to stop listening when someone is only half way through with his story or statement so that we may begin preparing our own. This is not listening and it always shows. Furthermore, there is no quicker way to negatively impact your interactions with others than to give an impression that you are not listening. To the other person, not listening is a sign that you don't think what they have to say is very important, or worst yet, that you don't think *they* are very important.

If you learn to listen well people may actually start following you around just because a good audience is so hard to come by. That is how rare an effective listener is. It is also why many individuals often pay therapists high hourly wages; just to have someone listen to their words, stories, and worries.

People are so unaccustomed to being truly heard that it may take them a while to accept that you are honestly an earnest listener. If you have posed your questions in the manner presented in the previous section, and in addition, actually hear the response, you will find yourself the most popular person at the party, in the boardroom, or at the beach. Everyone will want to talk to you because you identify with people as individuals, something people are begging for.

The act of listening itself is nothing revolutionary. You simply clear your mind, open your ears, and digest the words that are being transmitted your way. Think about what the other person has said. Swallow it. Sit with it. Don't rush to say something back. Listening is only effective if you've actually heard what's been said. When we respond too quickly, it's almost like we have failed to acknowledge what the other person said.

Another way to consider listening is to use your whole body. It shows when you're listening with your heart. Watch yourself in the mirror, look at how you appear when you are saying nothing but attempting to digest everything.

Have you ever been in a conversation where someone rolled his eyes when you spoke? How insulting was that? Or maybe more often, have you ever been in a conversation with another person, only to find them glancing at the paper, checking the time, or looking out the window? If you are not going to listen wholeheartedly, then do not give the illusion of listening at all; it is rude and ineffective. Many parents are guilty of this half-listening routine. Granted, children tend to talk often, and constantly seem to want our attention, but this is because they seek adult validation. If you have children, you should schedule a time each day when you can sit down, face to face, and talk about the day. Don't allow for any ringing telephones, television, or even rifling through of the mail. Make this your parent-child interacting time and keep it sacred.

Learning to listen with your body simply means that you are absorbing what is being said on a cellular level. You are drinking up the information and letting it rest inside before offering any kind of response. People will be impressed when you take the time to listen well. In addition to your own listening body language, consider the nuances related to those of the speaker.

People often speak to us with their bodies or their eyes. Sometimes, what they say with their words is not the same as what they say with their body. An obvious example of this is when someone greets you with closed arms and then methodically tells you that you are welcome to come inside. His body language clearly implies that you are unwelcome, yet the words of his discourse say otherwise. This requires deep listening and should not be ignored. Many times you can counter this contradictory message with good feedback, which will also be discussed in this chapter.

In the book, *How to Read a Person Like a Book,* which coincidentally was written by two litigation attorneys who are negotiation pros, body language is everything.
The authors give us some heads up on things to look out for, such as, when someone answers you affirmatively, but then scratches or rubs his nose, he really isn't sure at all. Another interesting one is that putting your fingertips together in the shape of steeple when speaking to others is a sign of confidence, while if you raise the steeple and peer through it, it is a sign of smugness.

Learning all about body language is time well spent. While there are ordinary body movements that we probably all have heard about, such as buttoning up your jacket and crossing your legs being signs of closing off, we often fail to consider them when we see them. When you speak to people or they speak to you, note important clues about how you come across to them and they to you. Open arms and hands indicate friendliness, while closed fists indicate frustration. People lean forward when they like an idea and pull back when they don't. A stroke of the chin means someone is sizing the situation up, and a touch of the lips usually means someone is holding something back.

While body language or eye contact may tell more of the story than the words alone, there is also the possibility that the speaker isn't fully aware of how he or she feels. While you can't expect to be a mind reader all of the time, there are instances when reading between the lines can take you farther into what's being said. When people are interacting, they sometimes overlook the emotional implications involved in the communication. If this happens, the other person might not even realize the issue and might not even be aware of what it is they're *not* saying. Again, the feedback tool is indispensable.

The feedback tool is a simple technology that assures you have completed correct listening skills. Offering feedback lets the speaker know that you have listened well enough to paraphrase back what has been said, and that you care enough to make sure your interpretation was correct. This tool can be very instrumental in accessing information that spans above and beyond what the speaker has said. First though, let's look at some examples of standard feedback that takes us closer to our goals.

You are a salesperson of photocopiers and you are trying to sell your product to Tyco Copy Center. You have had several visits with Mr. Gibbons and are now trying to close the deal.

> **You**: Well Mr. Gibbons, there you have it, a quality product at an affordable price.
> **Mr. Gibbons**: I don't know. I do recognize the quality... it's just that with an unknown brand....
> **You**: What is it about an unknown brand that makes you uncomfortable?
> **Mr. Gibbons**: I don't know, I mean, with our other machine if something went wrong, I'd just make a call.
> **You:** So, if I'm understanding you correctly, Mr. Gibbons, you'd like to be assured that our service department is as efficient and customer oriented as you've come to expect with the previous company. Is this correct?

When worded this way, Mr. Gibbons is likely to approve of the way the feedback was offered, agree with it, and then be convinced that it is true. When we really listen to what's being said, it becomes easier to repeat it in a manner that makes the speaker ever so impressed that they have been well heard. This is especially true when you have articulated the feedback even more clearly than it started out, such as the example above. This gives the other person the feeling that he has presented his opinion in a very eloquent manner.

Sometimes through effective listening we can assist people in better determining their own needs, even if those needs are different than initially assumed.

In this example, an employee we'll call James has asked to speak to his boss about a problem he's having with Janice, even though Janice isn't really the problem. It is only through his supervisor's astute listening and questioning skills that he is able to "hear" between the lines.

James: Thank you for seeing me.
Boss: Of course, what seems to be the problem?
James: It's the new girl.
Boss: Janice?
James: Yeah, Janice, she's been a real problem for me to work with.
Boss: Why's that?
James: It's the data entry, she does it all wrong and then I have to correct her mistakes.
Boss: How is she doing it all wrong?
James: Well she gets the shipping order first and then keys in separate.
Boss: And that causes mistakes?
James: Well, not exactly, but when I go to put my orders in, I'm working the regular way, and so I don't always see the purchase order number.
Boss: And then you make mistakes, because you're not accustomed to the number being in the second field.
James: Yeah! That's it exactly.
Boss: Have you talked to Janice about this?
James: Not exactly, but she's so headstrong, I can imagine she wouldn't pay any attention.

Boss: Well then, why not call her in right now and see if we can resolve this issue so that everybody is happy?

In this example Janice was new and hadn't even realized that inputting the purchase order first was causing so much frustration for James. While all conflicts might not be so easy to resolve, the point is that only through listening to what is being said, as well as what is not being said, are we able to fully understand the interaction at hand.

In the example above, the supervisor seemed to instinctively know that there was a miscommunication that had not been properly explored. If he would have simply stuck to the face value, not asking probing questions and listening intently, he might have interpreted an otherwise benign situation as an employee conflict, when no such conflict really existed. Part of listening, at least in theory, is the art of silence.

In her book, *Lions Don't Need to Roar,* Debra Benton tells us that silence is golden in corporate communications, "Both what you say and what you don't gets you to the top. Successful people know that. In fact, it seems as if the further up the corporate ladder, the fewer words they say." Men generally excel in this arena because, generally and historically, they always seem to have less to say, and perhaps this makes women nervous.

Women care about how everyone feels, what people are wearing, what kind of refreshments should be prepared, who's doing who, and a host of other matters that really rarely matter. We talk about losing five pounds, what happened last weekend, and what a pain in the you-know-what an ex-husband it. This is not to say we should change our natural tendency to communicate freely with our friends and loved ones. However, it is meant to imply that this craft of continual communiqué' should be curbed in those instances when a few minutes of quiet time might be just what the doctor ordered.

When a child, an employee, a superior or a partner comes to you, beyond making an effort to listen, learn to use the silence to your advantage. Whether it is buying you more time, giving you a chance to mull things over or allowing the other person time to compose, the silence can be a perfect segue into a more meaningful moment. As women, we seem driven to fill up empty space with something pretty.

Realize that this is just years of conditioning and that some walls look fine with nothing on them. There is power in silence.

Chapter Thirteen
IT'S TIME TO TALK

CONGRATULATIONS! If you have made it to this point you are well on your way to getting more out of your life by getting along better with the people in it. Once you start to understand and apply these techniques everyday, you will see how easy and amazingly effective it is. The good news is that this kind of action has a domino affect. When you are genuine in your communications with others are, they will usually follow suit. It stands to reason then that if enough people adopt these techniques, the whole world will begin to speak with a kinder tongue.

Now is the time to take everything we have talked about and put it into action. Here is where you respond to the situation in a manner that will be most effective in taking you toward your goal. This is what we've been building up to.

This section breaks up into several smaller sections. Each is intended as a vital piece of the puzzle. We will remember to remain calm, use words that are productive, keep a tone that is pleasing, make good eye-contact, use body language wisely and speak with confidence. We will also talk about the importance of applying the correct sensory style and building rapport with whomever we are communicating with.

Staying calm is often the most difficult thing of all. We hear something that doesn't set quite right with us and we forget everything we learned about stepping outside the situation, walking in the other person's shoes, asking questions and listening to answers. It will always present a challenge to remain completely calm about all things. Remember though, that people respond to what they see.

If you are dealing with someone and you react without thinking, chances are they will follow your lead. This is easily the most common cause of miscommunication. People fail to remain calm. Remaining calm presents a whole host of benefits, all worthy of consideration.

For starters, and right in line with the entire topic of this book, remaining calm makes you a much better communicator. Your interactions will always improve if you learn to keep calm. Even excitement that is something other than anger can be easily misconstrued. A rapid response, coupled with an adrenaline rush is the same physical reaction base as anger; the two can be easily confused. So even if you are excited in a positive way, or your frustration is aimed in another direction, be aware of how you are being perceived by others. People don't like to be yelled at or be the target for anger. When we fail to remain calm, we almost always enter into a non-productive mode.

Losing your cool rarely, if ever, accomplishes anything worthwhile. Losing your cool is never productive. Keeping your eye on the carrot can help you recall the importance of remaining calm. Remembering that you can never "unyell" at someone also helps. Finally, remaining calm avoids stress. Stress can kill you.

We've already touched on the negative impact that stress can have on your health. Therefore, it is vital to keep in mind that not remaining calm nearly always causes stress, even if it is only temporary. Also, losing your cool more likely than not will cause stress for the person you are losing your cool at. If both of you fail to remain calm, the stress that results from an out and out argument will make a hefty dent in your level of health for the day. Remaining calm can control the level of stress in virtually any interaction you might happen to encounter. Now seems a good a time as any to tell you about the kinds of negative physical reactions that stress can have on your body. This is particularly relevant because, as noted at the beginning of our journey, most all of our stress is in direct relation to our interactions with others. Short of being frustrated over a puppy you can't potty train or a baby who won't stay away from the china hutch, most all of your communications will be with people who are perfectly capable, in some way or another, of communicating with you, and it will be in the hub of these communications where you experience your most stressful encounters.

Here is a non-exhaustive list of diseases that have been either directly or indirectly attributed and/or linked to stress:

Heart disease
High cholesterol
Diabetes
Ulcers
Cancer (some forms)
Mental Illness
Immune Disorders and breakdown of (including AIDS)
Anxiety
Chron's Disease, Ulcerative Colitis, and Irritable Bowel Syndrome
Attention Deficit Disorder in children

Beyond this, which is already plenty to motivate us to avoid stress, when we fail to remain calm, we feel bad. When we lose our temper, or someone who we are talking to loses his temper, we feel a negative shift, emotionally and mentally. In addition to the physical and emotional stress, flared tempers in our interaction can make us wallow in self-pity, treat others unkindly, drink too much wine, or shrug off our remaining tasks of the day.

This isn't to say that there won't be times in your life when you lose your cool. Nor is it meant to imply that there won't be occasions when others lose their cool with you. Surely it affects us when someone speaks to us in a manner that we find distasteful, angry, disrespectful, or plain mean. The Big Rule to recall: **You can't change anything but yourself**. You can't change the fact that someone said something that was completely inappropriate. Maybe they lost their head and yelled when they should have whispered. Nevertheless, you have two choices subsequent to your response. And by the way, your response should be in accordance with the techniques we're discussing throughout this book.

You can either let it ruin your day, your week, your month, or you can write it off as someone else who has not yet mastered the art of effective communications. Then simply let it go. Why carry it around with you all day? Feeling bad won't change the weather and it won't

141

take the other person one inch closer to admitting he was wrong. Settle for taking solace in the fact that you have learned to rise above negative reaction, and aren't you glad? Instead of feeling rotten about someone else's misplaced rage and over reaction, think like this: *I have learned to respond instead of react and boy am I glad! Now that I see how bad it looks when someone reacts from their ego and insecurity; I realize how negative, draining and degrading it is, not to mention useless.*

Use those instances when others react negatively and hostile as little reminders of what *not* to do. Seeing it, even occasionally, provides ample opportunity to recall why *you* don't want to be like that. Moreover, and with respect to stressful communications and health, remember to take good care of yourself, both emotionally and physically. Above all, stay calm, and when someone else doesn't, overlook it as someone who has not mastered the art of interacting.

Part of understanding people is to know how to use the right words when you speak to them. Your word choice should avoid any accusatory connotations, yet be consistent and reflective of your position. When you employ smart word use, your interactions improve.

Perhaps the easiest way to remember productive word use is to never start your sentences with the word "you," if the sentence is going to be constructive or anything less than positive. When you start a sentence with the word "you," it almost always sounds like an accusation. This is not to say you can never start a conversation with the "Y" word. However, in conflicted communications or emotional interactions, it is a word best left behind.

Recall that during our discussion on negative reactions we talked about how people need to be right and how we all tend to get defensive when we feel that we are under attack. Starting a sentence with the word "you," in these instances is sure to evoke more of the same.

Avoid beginning any response by putting the other party in the hot seat; it's simply not effective. When you start a sentence with the word "you" in a conflicted communication the other party probably won't hear the rest of the sentence. They'll stop listening and begin reacting, and that's precisely what you want to avoid. To be most effective, you must take full responsibility for your actions and your position by using words that do not imply assumption.

Examine the different internal response or reaction in these sets of statements. Each "You" statement is followed with an "I" statement. Notice how the "You" statement sounds more accusatory, while the "I" statement seems to take responsibility. Consider the power this simple difference can have in your own interactions.

1. You make me feel like I'm wrong.
2. I feel that I may be wrong.

1. You gave me the wrong address.
2. I wrote down the wrong address.

1. You seem like you're mad.
2. I feel some tension.

1. You aren't giving me a chance to speak.
2. I feel like I'd like a chance to respond.

1. You need to slow down.
3. I feel like this is going too fast, can we back up?

1. You are not being clear.
2. I'm not getting this.

Do you see how changing the first word of each of sentence shifts the communication to a more productive mode? When you take responsibility in this manner, it doesn't mean you're assuming anything is your fault. It doesn't mean you are wrong or ignorant. Instead, it paves the way for improved interactions. It's important to remember that your ultimate goal is usually not to simply be right; if that's what you're after, join a debate club. In ordinary interactions, you'll want to check your ego at the door in order to get your point across in a way that doesn't seem overly offensive. Let the other person feel right sometimes— it will take you far.

The word "I" can be a tricky one. It's an excellent word for taking responsibility for your own interpretation because it avoids an accusatory connotation. Conversely, people are equally sensitive to self-centeredness.

Dale Carnegie tells us, "The New York Telephone Company made a detailed study of telephone conversations to find out which word is most frequently used. You have guessed it: It is the personal pronoun "I." "I" was used 3,900 times in 500 telephone conversations." Granted, this was written many years ago, but the point it makes is clear. People are often absorbed in their own perspective and position, and this can often be detected with an over usage of the "I" word.

So yes, taking responsibility for your tone and your message is vital, but remember to intersperse the use of the word "I" when you are interacting with others. Furthermore, while you're avoiding the act of calling excessive attention to yourself, notice those who do just the opposite and respond accordingly. People who consistently refer to themselves (as evidenced by over use of the word "I") in their interactions are often short on self-esteem. You can dramatically appeal to this in a positive manner by contributing, not detracting. Give the other person the lead. When someone wants to be a legend in his own mind, let him—- it's better than yelling and it gets you much farther.

We've already noted that people don't like to be yelled or shouted at. A word here about how you use your voice is warranted. Have you ever experienced someone speaking to you in a tone that you knew was less than sincere? Even worse, condescending? There is perhaps nothing more humiliating than to have someone speaking down to you. Keep this in mind when you are responding to others. Some people don't yell, they just assume a sarcastic tone, but this can be just as belittling as shouting outright. Treat people as you expect to be treated. Speak in a tone that is genuine and compassionate. Even on the phone, people can read your meaning if your tone is less than pleasing, supportive, or otherwise helpful.

There is at least one company who provides its customer service staff with a mirror right next to the telephone. The company wants its employee to remember to smile when they're on the phone. This is a smart company that recognizes its customers can "hear" a smile in the representatives' voice. Don't think that conversing over the wires, or even email for that matter, doesn't reveal tone. It does. A person can feel sincerity and enthusiasm in another person's tone. Be genuine.

While this book is primarily focused on oral communications, we live in an automated society where technology is becoming the norm in daily communications.

Even telephone communications are being replaced with emails, and those telephone calls that do get through often end up in voice-mail, leaving us to play a game we call "telephone tag." Telephone tag is an effective way to conduct a good deal of your business without ever having to talk to anyone. While it can surely be a convenient form of information transfer, it is a horrid way to improve your communication skills. There is nothing nearly as sincere as the human touch. Next time you leave a voice mail, ask yourself, do I need to leave all of the information, or can I just leave a message for the other party to call me back so I can give them the information "live?" Real time talking is far more effective than a recording. When you leave a voice mail message, speak slowly and confidently. Keep your tone upbeat and don't leave any more information that necessary. Many people make the mistake of talking into the receiver of voice mail as if the other person is really on the line, listening. This leaves the person who eventually retrieves the message bored beyond belief. Keep it simple, keep it short.

Say you wish to arrange to have a report proofread by an editorial firm. It is totally feasible to call the proofreader and leave him a voicemail message saying you'd like to drop off the work. He might call you back, leaving you a message this time, indicating that yes, please drop it off. You drop it off, then the next thing you know, he's leaving you a message saying you can pick it up; he'll leave it at the front desk. You might actually have an entire business transaction with someone without ever exchanging words "real time."

While living in the fast-paced world that we do, voice mail and electronic communications offer an excellent opportunity for streamlined communications. Americans tend to value saved time. For what reason, no one is sure. Getting so much done that you never have time to enjoy the journey makes little sense in other cultures, however, here at home, it's standard. If you're one of those people attached to your email and your cell phone at the hip, there are two rules worth remembering.

One, that you retain the same manner of communication consistency, although somewhat altered, regardless of the type of medium you are using. And two, that you don't allow the technologically advanced style of communicating to cause you to become rusty in real life. Face-to-face interactions with others will always have a place.

Also keep in mind that voice mail and e-mail do not allow for some of the "extras" that live interactions do. You must be twice as certain that the message you are typing (email) and talking to (voice mail), are well thought out and not subject to miscommunications. Exercise extreme care when using these short cuts of communications. And by all means, remember that there are some communications that are completely inappropriate when left in voice mail or presented via email. Important or sensitive information is better presented in person first, telephone second— not left as a message with no place for immediate response and discussion. Don't underestimate the value of direct interactions.

Direct interactions or face-to-face communications affords us the benefit of employing our body language in a productive way. Part of being genuine means that you put your whole body into your response. In the last section, we looked at body language as it relates to listening, now let's consider it from your perspective as the respondent, or speaker. The way you hold your body says a lot about the way you feel toward others, and even life itself.

Women especially, and unfortunately, have been grossly misconstrued over the decades simply by the clothes they choose to wear of they way they hold their bodies. This is clearly sad and unfair, however, a pound of prevention is worth a ton of cure. While we certainly are entitled to wear what we want to wear and act like we want to act, there are social constructs that must be permeated in order to excel in the corporate structure. Be smart and be observant. Notice what works and what does not. Be yourself, but always respect yourself for the person you are, and then, regardless of what you wear, the rest of the world will respect you too. Be true to your heart and you can't go wrong.

There are unfortunate stigmas in this society that are hard to kill. Add to that the continual barrage of new Bay Watch Babes clogging the filters and maintaining the status of what the rest of us try to change. It doesn't matter how you dress or how you hold your body. It's how you carry yourself, express yourself, treat yourself that really counts. Thank God for Erin Brokavitch. Beyond the feminine mystic, the importance of body language can be applied across both genders.

Do you stand with good posture? Good posture indicates honesty and self-esteem. Stand tall and you'll breathe deeper, another positive attribute. Do you gesture with your hands? People who put their whole body into their communications are often considered more sincere; beware though, too many movements can cause confusion and serve to distract your audience. If you move your hands at warp speed when you talk, you're going to take away from your message. Another form of body language that can be valuable in communications concerns mimicking. In NLP™ (neuro lingistics programming) mimicking is what we do to build instantaneous rapport with our audience.

Simply put, when you mimic someone (or "modeling" as it is often referred) you assume the same posturing, positioning, gesturing, tonality and range. The idea is that a person sees a reflection of himself in you, and that automatically makes him feel more comfortable in your presence, hence with you. Obviously this would best be applied in situations where you are dealing directly with one person or one group who is similar in their constructs. The caveat about mimicking is that discretion must be applied. Under no circumstances would you want the other party to think you are copying their every movement, as it might be interpreted as ridicule.

For instance, if you are talking to Bill, and Bill stands tall and proud, you too should assume a similar posture. If Bill faces you head on, you do the same. If, however, Bill tends to angle his body slightly to the right of yours, you stand in a way that compliments his direction. This kind of technique requires your attention. If Bill constantly pushes his hair back, you won't necessarily copy the exact same movement, however, you might casually reach up and rub the back of your neck for each time he rubs his head. Regulate your movements with his. Don't think of this as trying to be a mime downtown somewhere with your face painted white. Human interactions is very serious business and the idea of "modeling" has been studied extensively and proven to be an effective means of building instant rapport with other people. People simply feel more comfortable when they are dealing with those who seem to be like them.

Consider the strength this new knowledge might bring to all of your interactions, particularly your negotiations. People are much more agreeable if they like you. As a matter of fact, many people will bend over backwards and jump through hoops to make you happy, simply because they like you. They like you when they feel as if they have a rapport with you. When you mimic someone, you are paying them the highest compliment of all. You are saying, "You move and posture yourself like people are supposed to, and I am just like you, or at least want to be." What could be a greater compliment? People let their guard down and trust more easily when they are around their own kind.

Think about the last time you felt intimidated by someone. Perhaps they held their head up a little too high, or used their napkin differently and it made you feel like you were messy. Then, think about the times you've met someone you really liked, warmed right up to, maybe even someone who you were in awe of, a celebrity for instance. Didn't you utter the words, "He (or she) was so down to earth, just one of us?" The *"just one of us"* comment is the perfect definition of modeling. People respond to others who validate the way they are as being normal and acceptable. Remember this priceless technique and incorporate it when you are interacting with others.

Another way to relate better with others concerns their sensory style. Somewhat like modeling, the idea is that when you understand another person's style of perception, you can adjust your language to reflect that preference and build further rapport. Psychologists have long been aware that different people operate in strong association with one or more of their senses. Some people are more comfortable, or more compelled, to describe something based on one of the three senses; sight, sound, or touch. Those that lean toward the sense of sight, might use terminology such as, "The way I *see* things," or, "This *looks* like a big project." Sound-oriented people would say things like, "This project *sounds* like it will be big," or "If I'm *hearing* you right, this is what you're saying." Those who operate under the sense of touch, also known as kinesthetic, include "physically" related words such as, "I can't *get a handle* on this project," or "I *feel* like this is too big." Below is a brief list of words, as adapted from the book *Introducing NLP,* by Joseph O'Connor & John Seymour, that adds to the these categories. Listen for these words when you're dealing with others. Your key communications can benefit tremendously when you arm yourself with this information.

VISUAL KINESTHETIC	AUDITORY	
Outlook	Hear	Touch
Clear	Tone	Shock
Bright	Static	Tap
Clarify	Rattle	Crash
Graphic	Alarm	Push
See	Sound	Irritate
Show	Key	Grab
Reveal	Loud	Hit

There are of course, many other words that can be placed into each of the three categories. In some other countries that study sensory communications, the categories of scent and taste are added as well (something *smells* fishy, that leaves a bad *taste* in my mouth). You can learn something very important by this line of thinking. First, try and think about what kind of communicator *you* are. What terms do you use most of the time? Many people have a combination of two styles with one more predominate than the other. The reason this is important has to do with your ability to relate more easily and genuinely with another person. Learn to incorporate words from the other groups into your dialogue so that you ensure a universal impact, regardless of the audience.

Pay attention to the words other people use when they are talking. Take note as to which sensory style they most often apply and then match it. If your boss is largely an auditory speaker, make a "concerted" effort to incorporate auditory words into your diction. Tell him it "sounds" like a good idea. Let him know that the project is "crystal clear" and that you'll "compose" an email to that effect. When we speak in alignment with others, we build a much faster and stronger rapport. When a good rapport is developed, communications can proceed at a steady and progressive pace.

If you've ever noticed, people prefer to interact with those who possess a very similar style and level of articulation. This is precisely why some people refer to those with more expansive vocabularies as "snobs." This by no means suggests that you discontinue any attempts at expanding your vocabulary, but rather, be very observant as to the language-level of those you are interacting with, and then speak accordingly.

When we make an honest effort to mold our own communication style around the style of whomever we're talking to, we are handsomely rewarded. Besides building almost instant rapport, your interactions will be more productive. You cannot ask a person if he "comprehends" an idea if he never uses the word "comprehend" and may not be fully aware of its meaning. To match a person's vocabulary level and sensory style is courteous and effective.

It's no different than pulling out your Spanish handbook when you're on vacation in Mexico, or using hand motions to communicate with someone who is deaf; you are simply working on a level that makes the interaction more productive. If the other person doesn't get your meaning, you might as well be speaking pig Latin. Understand that building rapport with others will always be one of your most valuable assets— keep it well tuned.

Now let's talk about eye contact. Recognize right away how important it is to maintain eye contact. This is especially important for women who tend to appear less assertive than men; look 'em in the eyes if you want them to take you seriously. If you don't look someone else in his or her eyes, they won't take you seriously because they don't think you even take yourself seriously.

Above any other physical quality, good solid eye contact is inevitably the most important. Looking the person you are communicating with right in the eyes is vital to effective interactions. Even if you have to curl your toes to maintain eye contact, do it, never averting contact to look at the ground. Lowered eyes has long been associated with inferiority or shame, something we must work hard to alleviate in our new found communication skills. Beyond that, people won't respond positively if you don't maintain a certain level on eye contact.

Just think about it. Have you ever been in a class or seminar where the speaker was looking at his notes the whole time? Or perhaps he spoke to the ceiling, never making eye contact with the audience. We want someone to look at us when he's talking to us. It's validating to see that someone is directing his or her attention and words directly at us. While it's easier to deliver kind words with good eye contact, it is just as essential to make the same kind of eye contact with difficult or conflicted communications.

Obviously, there are times when we must be the bearer of bad news. Whether we are reprimanding an employee, informing an offspring they are grounded or telling a client the price went up, the way we communicate the news will certainly reflect upon our ability to interact well.

When you are delivering less than desirable information, eye contact is even more of a must. It might hurt to even think about it, but it counts here more than ever. When someone hears news that she doesn't necessarily want to hear, she's likely to react. By gaining and then holding eye contact, the person becomes much more connected to you, to your actions. For whatever reason, steady eye contact tends to soothe and reassure.

So if you must deliver news that might not be well received, always do it in person— not the telephone if it can be avoided—and never over email. Too many people have discovered that they can be brave in delivering criticisms and reprimands via email. It's not fair and it's certainly not effective. Don't say anything to anyone in writing or recording that you couldn't say right to his or her face. This is a critical to remember. Then, when you do meet face to face, make sure that you secure steady eye contact with the other person. Looking deeply into someone's eyes and sincerely expressing your sympathies can be genuinely helpful, regardless of the situation. In addition to lessening the blow, whatever it might be, you have positioned yourself in a role of authority, or at the very least, a role of someone who can communicate with confidence. The only caveat of this kind of eye contact worthy of mention concerns the proceeding section on modeling. Make every effort to mimic the level and degree of eye contact as the person you are interacting with.

For example, if Jennifer looks at you when she's talking, but only holds eye contact momentarily before talking to her hands, try to respond in a similar manner. This doesn't necessarily mean you have to talk to your own hands, but it does mean that you should be cognizant of Jennifer's preferred level of eye-contact-comfort, and act accordingly. Don't hold steady eye contact if it appears to make the other person uncomfortable, yet always make sure that they realize they are the focus of your attention. Steady eye contact usually denotes confidence and that it why it's wise to use.

There is an unmistakable line between ego and confidence. As we've discussed, ego operates from a lower level of insecurity and lack of self-esteem. The ego is generally selfish in its endeavors and feels like it's not getting its due reward. Self-confidence however, operates from the higher level of self-love and appreciation and allows a person to recognize the unique value she brings into the world.

A person who exudes self-confidence truly enjoys life. She may tend to have bad days like everybody else, but the main difference is that she never stays down for long. A person who has a self-confident attitude is always easier to talk to then a person who operates from pure ego, hands down. This is true because someone who feels good in her own skin can stop long enough to see the world outside. While on the other hand, the guy with an inflated ego is so uncomfortable and itchy, that he's barely able to take his mind away from his way of thinking and feeling. Who would you rather ask a favor of?

When you display confidence in yourself, you stand a much better chance at effective communications. People like people who like themselves in a healthy way. People with high levels of confidence, as contradictory as is may sound, are often more concerned with the well being of others, than their counter parts. If you think about this, it makes perfect sense.

Consider a person compelled by the need to be right. This person is probably suffering from an insecurity of some sort and uses his ego to cover it up. He will argue a point until he is blue in the face, just to prove he is right. He will criticize anyone who doesn't subscribe to his way of thinking. He probably loses his cool when someone doesn't get or support his point of view. Contrast this with healthy self-esteem.

The person operating with healthy self-esteem enjoys her life and her work. She probably likes to be around other people and explores other modes of thinking. Because she has respect for herself, respect for others is automatic. She won't interrupt you when you're speaking, she'll take responsibility for her own opinions but she'll be happy to listen to yours.

Which type of person would you rather interact with or even eat lunch with for that matter? Which one do you think would be quicker to help you overcome an obstacle? Who is going to listen to your concerns more compassionately? Who is the superior communicator? Self-confidence is truly the key to becoming the most effective kind of communicator you can. Just as you would prefer to interact with someone who had a healthy outlook on life, you must make the effort to see the world the same. When you feel good about yourself and others, people will knock down doors just to be around you.

In this section, we have discussed the physical qualities of responding effectively.

In addition to the words we use; the tone we use them in; and the way we manage our bodies; eye contact and self-confidence are all part of the master plan. In order to pursue the most productive communications, concentrate on incorporating all of these qualities into your tool box of talking and listening. Interact with your entire mind, body and spirit and you will see the world unfold before you. Now we will begin to consider the overall Theory in action.

In order to garner the most tangible benefits from ERT it is important that you consider it from each angle, both negative and positive. In the first example that follows, we will provide a conversation that has been based on negative reaction. For this particular study we will subsequently analyze the results as they relate to those we've previously discussed. Next, we will consider a revised version, this time applying the steps of the Effective Response Theory. It is important to understand that there are very few exacts in any social science. However, ERT is a guideline that will undoubtedly serve to improve all of your interaction skills when adopted and applied consistently. Remembering the primary component of keeping your goals in mind and then communicating toward them will take you far on this journey to productive communications.

After we review the two samples, we'll summarize with a comparison of productivity, attitude and health. As an extra bonus and opportunity for you to "show your stuff," there is a workbook that follows. See what you have learned.

As with any new theory, practice makes perfect. Now that you have read the background and application of this Theory, you'll need to determine how you might reduce it into simple and strategic steps that will be easy to automatically apply, regardless of the situation. Try it now.

The Case of the Missing File

Trudy is an administrative assistant with a chip on her shoulder. She's outgrown her position at the law firm where she works and there really isn't anywhere for her to go. She refuses to study to be a paralegal, even though the associates have offered to pay for the tuition.

Samantha is a newer attorney. She would like nothing more than to become a partner in the firm. She is much younger than the rest of the partners. As a matter of fact, she is the youngest person in the office. She is probably ten years younger than Trudy. Samantha is polite and friendly to everyone, but Trudy seems to have it in for her, at least that's how it feels. She doesn't give her messages as astutely as she does the partners in the firm, and she seems to be less friendly to Samantha then she is to the others.

The partners in the firm announce that Samantha will be given her first case. Samantha is ecstatic. Everyone in the office congratulates her, except for Trudy. Samantha spends extensive hours preparing for the case. She even prepares many of the papers and performs much of the research, just to ensure thing go smoothly the first day of court.

With the first day of the trial quickly approaching, Samantha asks Trudy if she would mind assisting her with some final papers. Trudy says she will, so Samantha leaves her the files and goes out to lunch. The next day, Samantha inquires about the papers and Trudy tells her she will be done by the end of the day. Samantha is relieved and figures she might have been a little pre-judgmental about Trudy; after all, she is helping her now.

The next day, Samantha, who is dressed professionally and ready for court, approaches Trudy and asks for the papers. Trudy assumes a blank look.

Samantha raises her voice: Don't tell me you lost them?

Trudy: I didn't lose them.

Samantha: Well you sat right there yesterday and told me they'd be ready.

Trudy: I know! And they were right here, under this stack.

Samantha: Jeez, I knew I should have done it myself.

Trudy: Listen, I did your papers, just like I said I would…

Samantha: Well a lot of good it did me. It's my own fault, I should have known.

Trudy: Known what?

Samantha: You've had it out for me since the beginning.

Trudy: Now you're talking crazy.

Samantha: Am I?

Trudy: Of course you are, I could care less about what you do or don't do.

Samantha: Yeah, that's why you lost my papers.

Trudy: That's it. I don't have to listen to your accusations!

Trudy spins around in her chair. She is seemingly insulted and refuses to give Samantha another moment of her time. Samantha finally has her day in court, with no papers and a bad feeling in her gut.

Let's look at what happened here.

First of all, even if Trudy was the one with the negative attitude, Samantha has the power to turn things around. Unfortunately though, Samantha became defensive at the first sign of a problem. Rather than probe into where the papers might be, giving Trudy the benefit of the doubt, Samantha jumped down her throat, accusing her of "having it in" for her.

In reality, Trudy was just plain tired of her job. She wasn't overly concerned with Samantha or with having her become too dependent on her support. It wasn't anything personal. Sure, she probably didn't like the fact that she was much younger than her, but it wasn't anything she lost sleep over. Samantha though, with the help of her own insecurities, made some exaggerated assumptions that cost her far more than she was willing to pay.

The interaction that took place with Trudy pulled Samantha farther from her goals, put her in a lousy mood, and the stress over the missing papers caused physical stress that made her feel ill. Was this a productive interaction?

Now let's apply the Effective Response Theory and see our plan in action.

Assume the same setting, same background.

The Case of the *Recovered* File

Trudy is an administrative assistant with a chip on her shoulder. She's outgrown her position at the law firm where she works, and there really isn't anywhere for her to go. She refuses to study to be a paralegal, even though the associates have offered to pay for the tuition

Samantha is a new attorney. She would like nothing more than to become a partner in the firm. She is much younger than the rest of the partners. As a matter of fact, she is the youngest person in the office. She is probably ten years younger than Trudy. Samantha is polite and friendly to everyone, but Trudy seems to have it in for her.

She doesn't give Samantha her messages as astutely as she does the partners in the firm, and she seems to be less friendly to her.

The partners in the firm announce that Samantha will be given her first case. Samantha is ecstatic. Everyone in the office congratulates her, except for Trudy. Samantha spends extensive hours preparing for the case. She even prepares many of the papers and performs much of the research, just to ensure thing go smoothly the first day of court.

With the first day of the trial quickly approaching, Samantha asks Trudy if she would mind assisting her with some final papers. Trudy says she will, so Samantha leaves her the files and goes out to lunch. The next day, Samantha inquires about the papers and Trudy tells her she will be done by the end of the day. Samantha is relieved and figures she might have been a little pre-judgmental about Trudy; after all, she is helping her now.

The next day, Samantha, who is dressed professionally and ready for court, approaches Trudy and asks for the papers. Trudy assumes a blank look.

First of all, following the intuitive steps of ERT, Samantha has already identified her goals:

> ➤ **Long-range goal**: to become a partner in the firm
> ➤ **End-goal**: to win this case
> ➤ **Mini-goal**: to find the missing file

Next, she'll *step outside of the situation* and assess only the facts:

1. She said she'd help me.
2. I've got to go to court in 20 minutes
3. The files are missing

Now, she'll quickly *empathize* with Trudy. She might indeed be a little jealous, in which case some reassurance could be helpful. She probably is tired since it's the billing time of the month, and might respond to a little support. Samantha then proceeds with asking *useful questions.*

Trudy: I thought they were right here.
Samantha: Hmm, could they be under a stack of invoices?
Trudy: I don't think so, but let's look.

Trudy begins getting frantic as she explores her desk. Samantha *remains calm and confident, demonstrating her unwavering faith in Trudy:*

Samantha: I hate it when I do that- I was notorious for it in law school, I swear my files just grew legs and walked away. (Samantha attempts to lesson the burden for Trudy, showing her that she supports her. This is highly effective in these situations.)
Trudy: I finished them at about 7:30— that I know for sure.
Samantha: Wow, I didn't realize you had to stay so late to get them done.
Trudy: No big deal…I got it! The copy room, I'll bet I left the whole file in the copy room because I was waiting for the copy machine to warm up.

Sure enough, when Samantha and Trudy venture into the copy room, the pile of perfectly prepared papers are sitting right there. Samantha is just in time to head off to court, thanking Trudy on her way and letting her know she's got a free lunch coming.

By following the steps Samantha was able to find her papers and all's well that ends well. Once again, let's review and briefly summarize the steps of the Effective Response Theory.

1. **State your purpose**. Identify your long range, short-range, and immediate goals. Knowing where you need to go takes you far in getting there. By constantly focusing on your goals, you are much more likely to act in alignment to them. Remember that long-range goals are the ultimate goals you are working toward, your end goals are the goals of most general communications and the ones that take you toward your long term goals, and your mini goals are those little cogs in the wheel that we all contend with.

2. **Step outside the situation**. Strip your emotional involvement and simply state the facts in a congruent manner. It will help you better assess the real issue at hand, while allowing you to see the next most logical step. Remember, there is no room for emotion, judgment or suspicion in this step of the Theory—just the facts please.

3. **Walk in their shoes**. Learning to empathize is one of the most important skills in your arsenal of interaction tools. Understanding how other people see things and how they might be feeling gives you extra insight. It also helps you to remember that you are dealing with someone who, just like you, has a vested emotional interest in the interaction. Empathize often.

4. **Ask and Listen**. Learn the art of effective questioning. Smart questions are ones that lead to answers that take you closer to your goal. Listening means hearing what the other person is saying. Remember to listen fully to all forms of communication, including body language and unvoiced concerns.

5. **Respond**. Before you even open your mouth, ask yourself the 64 million-dollar- question: *Will this bring me closer to my goal?* Then, remember to speak productively, with a calm demeanor and a kind tone. Recall the benefit of building rapport by modeling the other person's stance and diction. Exude positive body language and energy, make constant eye contact and maintain a sense of self-confidence.

Using the example of Samantha and Trudy, let's look at a comparative analysis between Negative Reaction and Effective Response Theory.

<u>**Negative Reaction**</u> vs. <u>**Effective Response Theory**</u>

Was the interaction
Productive?   NO!   YES!

Did the communication Result in an improved attitude?	NO!	YES!
Did the communication cause Physical stress?	YES ☹	NO! ☺

These are the three vital questions you should always remind yourself of prior to an important interaction, and then check with yourself afterward to see if they were satisfied. Whatever kind of unique shorthand you devise to keep them in mind is fine, but you will find that these are the three critical components, or guide-posts, to effective communications.

Your interactions should:
o   Be Productive
o   Improve or maintain a positive attitude for both parties
o   NOT cause undue physical, emotional or mental stress

If you can manage to keep these qualifications in mind prior to critical communications, negotiations, sales calls, interpersonal conversations, debates, and daily dialogue, you will be well on your way to the cutting edge of communications. It doesn't matter if you're confronting an employee, calling your mother after an intense argument, applying for a new position, disciplining a youth or simply trying to clear up a misunderstanding with the phone company, these are sure-fire steps to ensure you come out a winner every time.

Now it's your turn to apply this technique in a few different situations. You will be guided through the steps. Complete the sentences as you deem appropriate for the scenario at hand. Please do not skip this portion of the book. We often assume that once we've read and understood something we can file it away for future use. It doesn't always work like that. Repetition is the mother

Through this kind of applied guided practice you will learn to automatically apply the Theory quickly and easily. Once it becomes mentally ingrained, little effort will be required on your part. These exercises have been carefully crafted to assist you in automating the process. Please do not skip them.

After you have completed the first set of exercises, new ones follow that will require you to apply situations more common in your own personal and professional life. Again, it is only through careful and frequent self-exploration that we can begin to understand ourselves. Through such understanding, we are better equipped to harness and direct our potential reactions and our effective interaction efforts.

Exercise

Situation: You have been talking to a client who has all but accused you of lying. This is a client you have worked with for several months now and you've not known him to ever be this aggressive. You suspect he has somehow been misinformed about the new billing procedure, but nevertheless, he's taking it out on you. You are trying to win salesman of the month award and do not want to lose his business. He says to you, "I don't think you even appreciate my business, and this new billing system you guys have is really screwing my books up."

Your Goals:
Long term: _____
Immediate:_____
Mini:_____

Step outside the situation…what do you see? Note only the facts:

_____
_____
_____

Walk in the other person's shoes:

_____
_____
_____

Ask Questions/Listen:

_____
_____
_____
_____
_____
_____
_____
_____

Respond effectively (make sure what you say brings you closer to your goal):

_____
_____
_____
_____
_____
_____
_____
_____
_____
_____

Exercise

<u>Situation</u>: You are promoted to the new position of Creative Coordinator where you oversee all the advertising that comes out of the company. The junior position is held by Jerry, someone who applied, and was hoping to gain the position you just got. The end of the first month, when an important ad campaign is scheduled for release, you note that Jerry has not fulfilled his responsibility. You try and hedge the issue by inquiring when he thinks he might have his part of the project complete. Jerry snaps, "If I'm not working hard enough for you, why don't you just fire me?"

Your Goals:
Long term: _____
Immediate:_____
Mini:_____

Step outside the situation…what do you see, facts only?

_____

_____

Walk in the other person's shoes:

_____

_____

Ask questions/Listen:

_____

_____

Respond effectively (make sure what you say brings you closer to your goal):

Exercise

Situation: Your partner has been working many late hours. You're a little irritated that things around the house haven't been getting done, but you realize it's a very busy time at work for your partner, so you try to be understanding. Then, you notice that a late bill from the utility company comes stating that your electricity will be turned off in 24 hours if the bill is not paid. This is something your partner said had already been done the week prior. How do you approach this?

Your Goals:
Long term: _____
Immediate:_____
Mini:_____

Step outside the situation…what do you see, facts only?

_____

_____

_____

Walk in the other person's shoes:

_____

_____

_____

Ask questions/Listen:

_____

_____

_____

Respond effectively (make sure what you say brings you closer to your goal):

_____

_____

_____

In each of these exercises you were asked to identify the goals of concern. Clearly, in your own experiences, there may or may not be a long-term goal to consider, such as staying married or keeping your job, that you'll want to consistently hold in your mind. So consistently in fact, that you should remind yourself of it each time you enter any interaction with any party who is relevant to that goal. Beyond that, the exercises were fairly self-explanatory.

The "Respond Effectively" section left space for you to compose an acceptable statement in response to the overall interaction. The statement should have been conducive to a positive and affable outcome that satisfied our three primary areas of interest: productivity, attitude and stress. While it wasn't necessary to write, it is important to recall that part of responding effectively requires we assume a pleasant tone, pleasing body language, frequent eye contact and a confident demeanor.

Now it's your turn to get a little more personal with what you've learned. Use the following three exercises to create and respond to situations you have *already* experienced that caused some kind of grief because the interaction went haywire, or, one that might be quite likely in your life. This exercise will be most effective if you can recall or create scenarios that tend to tap your unique triggers—the ones that make you crazy. Further, note in the "Goals" section, a life-goal has been added so that you may insert whatever overall goal you have that is be relevant to that particular interaction.

Finally, to gain the absolute most from these exercises be sure to include both personal and professional situations.

Situation:

_____
_____
_____
_____
_____
_____
_____
_____
_____
_____
_____
_____

Goals:
Long term: _____
Immediate:_____
Mini:_____

Step outside the situation…what do you see, facts only?

_____
_____
_____

Walk in their shoes:

_____

_____
_____

Ask questions/Listen:
_____
_____
_____

Respond effectively (make sure what you say brings you closer to your goal):
_____
_____
_____
_____
_____
_____

#2
Situation:
_____
_____
_____
_____
_____
_____

Goals:
Long term: _____
Immediate:_____
Mini:_____

Step outside the situation…what do you see, facts only?
_____
_____
_____

Walk in their shoes:

_____
_____
_____

Ask questions/Listen:

_____
_____
_____

Respond effectively (make sure what you say brings you closer to your goal):

_____
_____
_____
_____
_____
_____
_____
_____

#3
Situation:

_____
_____
_____
_____
_____
_____
_____
_____
_____

Goals:
Long term: _____
Immediate:_____
Mini:_____

Step outside the situation…what do you see, facts only?

_____
_____
_____

Walk in their shoes:

_____
_____
_____

Ask questions/Listen:

_____
_____
_____
_____
_____
_____

Respond effectively (make sure what you say brings you closer to your goal):

_____
_____
_____
_____
_____
_____
_____
_____
_____

Chapter Fourteen
IT'S ABOUT BEING NICE

YES, There is an Art to Being Nice.

In spite of all the steps and processes that might be attributed to psychology and communication theory, it all really boils down to this: if we want to get along well with others and be well liked, we need to be nice. There are some brilliant authors of the past who have laid this out in terms so simple that even a fourth-grader could understand them. It does not require a doctoral degree or knowledge of nuclear physics to grasp the basic secrets of how we can get along better in the world and with the people in it. Some of these authors, such as Napoleon Hill, Dale Carnegie, Og Mandino and others, stated for us in easy to understand terms the obvious and evident facts about people.

Let's take a look at some of these age-old premises with a set of modern eyes.

1. **Don't criticize, whine, complain, or belittle**. This couldn't be an easier one to understand. Be impeccable with your speech, especially as it relates to others. Don't gossip or antagonize someone simply because you can. This includes children and people who are in subordinate positions. When you realize that all of the time and effort you spend talking about other people is nothing more than negative energy you are expending and creating, you will learn to keep your mouth closed. The adage that your mother once taught you, "If you can't say anything nice, say nothing at all," is especially true today, in all modes of communication.

We are all allotted a particular amount of energy that we are able to spend each day. Just like our bank account or vacation days, when we use it up, it's gone. Once you grasp this idea, and recognize that your energy can escalate to the next level, simply by uttering kind words instead of condemnations, you will see a better way to live. Reclaim your right to conduct yourself each day with an abundance of energy by refraining from negative talk. Speak well to and of others, period.

"What about venting?" someone once asked, does venting about a boss, co-worker or neighbor count as complaining? You bet. Let's consider the intent behind venting. Say your neighbor parks in front of your house and it really bothers you. Say it doesn't bother you enough to mention it to him, but it bothers you plenty enough to mention it to your room mate. You may rant and rave and kick the door for a few minutes. Once you gather your senses and straighten your posture, you might even note that you were merely "venting," but you feel better now. First of all, how much better do you reckon your room mate is feeling?

Negative energy is negative energy no matter how much you try to dress it up. Contrary to popular belief, "venting" doesn't do anything positive for your emotional well being, and it certainly doesn't do anything for those who you are venting in front of or to. When we vent, what we are really doing is asking someone else to agree with us that so and so is wrong and we are right. Doesn't this sound a lot like the ego at work?

If something or someone is bothering you, forget about venting simply for the sake of complaining to an audience who you expect to agree with and feel sorry for poor you. Instead, approach whatever the situation is with a level head. Consider what part of the circumstance you might be taking much too personally (or seriously, for that matter). Then ask yourself if this is one of those earth shattering revelations that deserves immediate military interaction or rather, is it something that you should just let roll off your back for now? Learn to recognize those things in your life that you cannot live with and change them— accept the rest without complaint. Remember to apply the previous steps in conflicted or challenging communications to strive for more wholesome interactions.

2.   **People love to hear their own name**. As a matter of fact, some of us would call their own name one of the prettiest

they've ever heard. Good salespeople, since the beginning of time, have known this truth, yet many of us fail to apply it in a manner that helps us reach our goals. How many parents only address their children by full name when the child is in trouble or acting up? When is the last time you have uttered your lover's name, for no reason at all? Do you say the names of co-workers as you greet them each day? Don't under- estimate the power of names when you're speaking to clients and employees.

Most likely, it comes from the fact that our name is one of the single unique qualities we can claim as our own. When people use it, it reminds us of how very unique we are. It keeps us individualized from the rest of the world. It is not uncommon, based on baby-name trends that seem to continue throughout the decades, that you might find yourself working in a situation with two or more people sharing the same name. In this case, it is still essential to further separate the two so that each can remain unique. For example, in an office with a Jennifer Jacobs and a Jennifer Harmon, ask them each what they prefer to be called. Perhaps one would like to be known as Jenn or Jenny, or maybe the name and the first initial of the last name, such as "JennJ." Never underestimate the power behind someone's name.

3. **Make people feel important**. It doesn't matter if you have to bite your tongue when someone says they just went skiing, and you did the Alps only a month ago. Keep quiet. Give the other person a moment in the spotlight and he or she will never forget you for it. People need to shine. They need to know that they are important and that their accomplishments are worthy of your time and attention.

Often times you will find people saying things that cause you to put up a big red flag over their head. You'll recognize immediately the weaknesses in other peoples' communication skills. You'll note to yourself, "Ah, he is very insecure to say that," or, "She clearly needs to have her ego tended to, having made that kind of remark." When these instances stand out to you, it means two things. First, that you have truly gained an understanding of human nature and the nuances of effective interactions. Secondly, and assuming that you didn't *react* to the statement, it shows that you have learned to apply these techniques toward much more productive and effective communications.

When you learn to let other people feel important, you hold the world by its axis. There is no quicker way to rise to a superior level of existence than to let other people feel as important as they need to feel. It doesn't matter if their claim to fame is nothing more than an illusion of grandeur. It doesn't matter if the attention they are calling to themselves is nothing more than a way to make them feel good about themselves when an unhealthy self-esteem is obvious. What does matter is your ability to overlook the obvious and not let yourself get riled up by the temptation to react.

If John said he was the fastest runner at the company ball game, and you know for certain it was Kate, or worse yet, you, who cares? Remember what we said earlier; ask yourself, will the truth have any relevance on your life as you know it? Will putting John in his place do one single thing to improve your interactions with him? Of course not. And who cares? This isn't about learning to make enemies; people already tend to fare quite well in that area. Take solace in the fact that you know the truth and save your energy for bigger and better battles. This is about letting others be legends in their own mind, assuming that the scenario has no tangible detrimental impact on you or others.

Understanding ego and insecurities in yourself and others is vital to effectively allowing others their moments of glory. Realizing that nothing will change if you let John say and think he was the fastest runner at the ballgame is to your advantage. Furthermore, recognize how much damage would be caused if you aptly pointed out to John that he ran slower than your toddler. While you might experience a fleeting moment of "one up," John would find you highly egotistical, insecure, and a lousy communicator. Even worse, if anyone else is listening to the conversation, they will think the same. Is it really worth it? Not even for a second. Let the other person feel important— even help them get there.

4. **Let people come up with ideas on their own**. As a matter of fact, let them take credit for those ideas you helped them discover. People are much more agreeable toward taking action on ideas that they assume ownership of. You will find if you ask intelligent questions, listen well, and repeat what you hear, that people can often create their own solutions to problems, or ideas for excellence.

    As an example, say you were trying to sell an insurance plan to a nice couple with one child. Rather than tell them that if they don't have insurance and something happened to one or both of them, their child would be financially doomed, start out by asking them questions that allow them to form their own conclusions. You might preface your question with a compliment such as, "I can tell your family is important to you. What kind of plans are you considering for college? She sure looks like an ambitious little thing." Here, you have given the couple credit by letting them know you already see they are caring people. Next, you've posed the casual question about college, followed again by a compliment that confirms the obvious (an ambitious child).

    The couple can come up with their own conclusion. They might think, yes, she will need college funds, of course she will, and what if...what if something happened to us...how could we be sure she'd have the money to go to college or be cared for? The couple will soon enough conclude that life insurance is a good idea, but please note, it was their idea, not yours.

5. **Do favors for others**. It takes some of us a lifetime to realize that the best part of living is the gifts we impart unto others.

When people get caught up in their own success they often fail to see the value in simple acts of kindness. It isn't always about closing the deal or getting the raise. It isn't always about winning the game or proving your point. We have created a results-oriented society where sometimes a coffee break seems out of the question, let alone carrying out favors for friends (or strangers, no less!).

The point is simple. Everything you do in life will come right back at you...eventually. If you are selfish or thoughtless to someone else, go ahead and plan to receive the same kind of treatment, some day, some way. What comes around goes around. That is reason enough to avoid bad behavior toward others. We noted before how important it was to see things from the other person's point of view-- this is along the same lines. If you always remember to walk in the other person's shoes, you'll get a lot less blisters. Learn to be of service to others.

Conversely, when you do good things for other people or causes, with no motive other than to just be nice or bring a little sunshine to the world, the favor will come back at you, often many times over. There are a couple of caveats worth noting here. First of all, when you do something great, like rescue a friend with a flat tire; give a million dollars to the University; or volunteer to organize the company holiday dinner, don't call attention to yourself. The bible actually mentions the fact that people who call attention to their good deeds get their rewards from the attention they receive, while those who say nothing, have greater things coming. Of course that's not the exact terminology used in the bible, but the meaning is the same: brag about how nice you are and don't expect much beyond a pat on the back or a rolling of the eyes.

On the other hand, when you do something really great for someone else, under the very guises of doing it and expecting nothing in return, your rewards will be on-going. It might take days, weeks or even years, but you will somehow, some way be repaid for your unselfish acts of giving. Clearly this requires a little faith above and beyond what is considered basic, but it is faith well vested.

6. **Expect the best in others**. When you enter into a conversation, sale, negotiation, objection or conflict, arm yourself with magic. Always go in thinking that the other person is just as smart, just as worthy and just as noble as you. Something about our expectations can cause us to act in a way that make them seem true, and before we know it, they are true. If you expect the valet to park your new car with extreme care, and you let him know you trust that he will do just that, chances are he won't let you down.

    It's been noted time again how children who are raised with a certain degree of discipline are happier and better adjusted. Discipline, in its most basic sense, is nothing more than investing faith in a child that the rules will be kept and that you will enforce them as necessary. The kids might mess up every now and then, just to make sure you're watching, but generally speaking, children respond to great expectations.

    This is the same in adulthood. When people have faith in us, think we are capable and able, we will work twice as hard to prove them right and to win their approval. Have no faith that your employee can complete his project on time, and then watch him fail. Take the same employee and let him know you're betting on his effort, and watch him succeed. People respond to the expectations of others.

    When you hold high expectations that the person you are interacting with has the same level of integrity, honesty and good intention as you do, you will help to inspire and encourage those exact traits in her or him. Go into the situation letting the other person know, however discreetly, that you recognize these are qualities the two of you share. You will be amazed at how people rise to the occasion to act with honor. And, you will be delighted at how much more productive your interactions are when your start out from a positive place.

7. **Air your own mistakes, cloud theirs**. When dealing with other people we've already noted that the ego has the floor. The worst thing you can do is to call attention to the other person's mistakes. Because of our egos and insecurities, we always are on the lookout for someone who might be implying that we're somehow not up to par; pulling our weight; or the cause of the fiasco. Sometimes, we're so busy worrying about those petty matters, that we miss the big picture, and that can really play havoc with productive communications.

   The best way around this from the get go, is to note your own errors. Yes, it takes a confident person to point out her own mistakes, but it also produces a person who knows how to get things done. After all we've learned about the ways ego and insecurity skew our communications, this should be easy enough to swallow. When you note the mistakes you've made in the past, you do two things.

   First, you let the other person know that you yourself are not perfect. What a relief that can be for any one; not needing to worry about how to act in the presence of perfection. Secondly, if you've done your job well, you've unarmed defensive behavior so that the matter at hand can be better addressed. When you do bring forth someone else's error, cloud it up a bit. Avoid accusatory statements and a general sense of negativity. For example, while you might come right out and tell Ralph that he messed up the order and that now you've got seven sides of beef with no freezer room, you've got to wonder how effective that's going to be. First, Ralph is going to be consumed in anger and defensiveness over your accusation. Maybe he has an excuse, maybe not. The point, however, is that you want a solution to the problem of all that potentially wasted meat, not a sonnet of explanations from Ralph. Since your immediate goal is to get the problem resolved in the most productive manner possible, consider your approach.

   Blatantly accusing Ralph and demanding action *might* get you a quick, albeit sloppy solution. In an effort to make sure the job is done well and your relationship with Ralph maintained, think about alternative approaches. If you preface the communication with empathy, perhaps even recalling an incident when you made an error in judgment, Ralph will hold a healthier perspective and be much more receptive to your needs.

Transform a problem into a situation that requires his assistance, not a mess that he needs to fix. People are often best held accountable when you let them come forward on their own. Of course, this isn't always applicable, but in common blunders, it works well. With Ralph, note there was on over order on the beef and now you need his help in resolving it. Even if it is not his mistake, he will be more than willing to take ownership in resolving the problem, simply from the way it was presented.

Even later, if any kind of reprimanding in required, recall that adults, like children, respond well to rules that are reinforced. They respect authority, however, treat them less then adequate or noble, and that is precisely what you will receive. This doesn't necessarily mean that if you're a manager, a CEO, or the president of a company, you should go around telling the company how many bad deals you've been responsible for. There is a certain amount of respect you'll need to carry around as the leader of the pack. However, don't ever underestimate the power of being human.

People respond strongly and supportively to those leaders who present themselves as human beings first, bosses second. Admitting that you've exercised poor judgment a time or two can do more good than harm. Furthermore, when you show others your perseverance, your ability to pick yourself up and continue in spite of the roadblocks is when you're wearing your leadership suit in full color.
Let's summarize this chapter on the basic rules of the road for being nice, remember them, copy them, paste them on your mirror or next to your computer—they will serve you well.

1. **Don't criticize or complain**. People don't want to hear negativity, even when they are full of it themselves. Maintain a pleasant demeanor. Avoid gossiping at all costs and avoid those

who tend to drain your energy by talking negatively about others, or complaining in general.

2. **Use a person's name when you speak.** People love the sound of their own name and to incorporate it in your speech will give you instant credibility and help build rapport.

3. **Help other people feel important**. As we have noted throughout, people love to be the star and shine in their very own movie. In life, let others take the leading role when it comes to having the spotlight. Nothing makes your own light shine brighter.

4. **Help people form ideas, and then give them the credit for it**. Whether you're selling a house, a car or an idea, when you let the other person come to conclusions on her or his own, the idea will be more appealing. Help people come to the conclusions you are working toward, and then congratulate them for their intelligence.

5. **Do favors for others, or secret acts of kindness.** It might be something as small as a phone call or something as time consuming as a full day of volunteer work. When you are of service to others, with no ulterior motive, the favors will multiply many times over and be returned to you, often when you least expect it. Be nice simply for the sake of being nice. Take time to help others without them always having to ask first.

6. **Expect the best in others and that's just what you will get**. When you walk into in interaction with an attitude of gratitude, anticipating wonderful things, that's usually what you'll get. Think about it. When you walk into a room, worried about the negotiation, what usually will usually ensue is the very issues you concerned yourself with. Expect good things of others and they will bend over backwards to see that you get them.

7. **Air your own mistakes; be constructive with the mistakes of others**. We're usually so busy hiding our errors and calling attention to the errors of others that we seldom take time to consider the damage we are doing. By simply admitting your mistakes and being constructive in the feedback toward the mistakes of others, you have made yourself an all-time hero. People will love you for brushing over boo boo's, especially when you are first to admit your own.

These time-tested ideas, when applied faithfully, will change your world.

Conclusion

THIS book has provided you with enough information that you could spend the rest of your life perfecting it. Indeed, if you simply learned to apply a percentage of these techniques into your day-to-day interactions, you would improve your ability to get along in life and with others at least a hundred-fold. There is no doubt that in our communications we hold the key to success, happiness, and longevity. The way we conduct ourselves now, matters more than ever.

Gender differences are also at an interesting crossroads. Women and men are still, in some ways, in the dark ages when it comes to communications. However, there are thru-ways as never before, and opportunities for increased awareness, understanding, and cooperation.

Women today can run companies, cities and nations. We can bake bread, paint portraits, raise children and raise cane. We can start our own businesses, find and pursue our deepest passions, and take the world on, head first. The time has come when we must cull all of our strengths and be the people we were meant to be. If you want to wear dresses and smell pretty, do it. If you prefer jeans or wearing a tie, that's okay too. The point is that we no longer need to worry about fitting into someone else's ideology of what a woman is, or what she should strive to be. With this, comes responsibility.

Now that the playing field is attempting to level itself out in some ways, (at least more ever before), we can begin to get back in touch and in tune with our deeper selves; our intuitive, loving, caring, creative selves that have been hindered throughout the centuries. This book is about putting this modern demeanor into action. It is not to say that men shouldn't read and apply these techniques. They should. It is instead to say that there must be gender balance, and gender balance begins with the way we interact with others.

These are not secret formulas or magic potions. These are fail-proof techniques that will help you get ahead. We cannot progress in this world without the assistance and compliance of others; it is just not possible. Use your inherent intuition, compassion and common sense when dealing with other people. Bring confidence and clarity into all of your interactions, discarding ego-infested defenses in yourself, and overlooking them in others, and the light is sure to spread.

It is my sincere wish that the people who read and apply the proven techniques within these pages will rise miles in their happiness and success, while finding all relationships and interactions more empowered than ever before.

Bless you!

Bibliography

Alessandra, Tony, PH.D, & Hunsaker, Phil, PH.D. *Communicating At Work.* New York: Simon & Shuster, 1993.

Benton, DA. *Lions Don't Need To Roar.* New York: Warner Books, 1992.

Bramson, Robert, PH.D. Coping With Difficult People. New York: Dell, 1981.

Brinkman, Rick, Dr. & Kirschner, Rick, Dr. Dealing With People You Can't Stand.
New York: McGraw-Hill, 1994.

Carnegie, Dale. How To Win Friends & Influence People. New York: Pocket Books, 1936.

Carlson, Randy & Leman, Keven, M.D. Unlocking The Secrets of Your Childhood Memories. New York: Pocket Books, 1989.

Carter, Les, Dr. & Minirth, Frank, M.D. The Anger Workbook. Nashville, TN: Thomas
Nelson Publishers, 1993.

Fisher, Ronald P., & Ury, William. Getting to Yes: Negotiating Agreement Without Giving In. Boston: Houghton Mifflin, 1981.

Hill, Napoleon. Grow Rich! With Peace of Mind. New York: Fawcett Crest, 1967.

Leeds, Dorothy. The Seven Powers of Questions: Secrets to Successful Communications in Life and at Work. New York: Penguin Putnam, Inc., 2000.

Littlejohn, Stephen, W. Theories of Human Communication. New York: Wadsworth Publishing Company, 1999.

Mandino, Og. The Greatest Salesman In The World. New York: Bantam Books, 1968.

Nierenberg, Gerard, & Calero, Henry. How to Read a Person Like a Book.

O' Connor, Joseph, & Seymour, John. Introducing NLP. London: Thorsons, 1990.

Reeve, Johnmarshall. Understanding Motivation and Emotion. Second Edition. New York: Harcourt Brace College Publishers, 1997.

Seligman, Martin, E.P., PH.D. Learned Optimism: How to Change Your Mind and Your Life. New York: Pocket Books, 1990.

Sternberg, Esther, M. M.D. The Balance Within- The Science Connecting Health and Emotions. New York: Freeman, 2000.

Vaughn, Susan, C., M.D. Half Empty Half Full: Understanding the Psychological Roots of Optimism. New York: Harcourt, 2000.

The Levinson Letter, The Great Book of Business Secrets, Boardroom Classics, New York, The Working Communicator, Sample Issue, Decemeber 14, 2000.

Communicating Better at Work, Communication Breifings. Voume XIX. No.1 Virginia.

"Catching" a Happy Mood, Roland Neumann, Ph.D. Woman's World, Volume 16, January, 2000.

About the Author

*T*AMARA Dorris is a writer, coach, and college professor in Sacramento, California, where she lives with her husband, Greg, her four kids, Nichole, Kelly, Jessica, and Kyle, her two dogs, Sage and Missy, two cats, Cosco and Crisco, a box turtle, and a rabbit who thinks he's girl.

*T*AMARA does college and corporate workshops, and consulting. She can be reached at Tamara2@surewest.net or at Empowered Press Publishing 916.482.5834.

Printed in the United States
33314LVS00006B/373-420